Health On Demand
Nurturing The Universe Within

7 Strategies to Optimize Your Health
& Prevent Chronic Illnesses

Solanyi Ulloa

7 Strategies to Optimize Your Health & Prevent Chronic Illnesses.

Health on Demand
Nurturing the Universe Within
By Solanyi Ulloa

Published by Garden of Neuro Publishing
A Division of the Garden of Neuro Institute
Poughkeepsie, New York
www.GardenofNeuroPublishing.com
Copyright © Solanyi Ulloa

ISBN eBook 978-1-962077-03-3
Cover Design Solanyi Ulloa

Table of Contents

"Health is the greatest of human blessings."
Hippocrates

Preface

Welcome to Health on Demand (HOD), a comprehensive book empowering you to take charge of your health and well-being. Everyone deserves access to the knowledge and resources essential for leading a healthy, joyful life. Within the pages of this book, you will discover invaluable insights to make informed decisions about your health. It will serve as a compass on your wellness journey, providing actionable information to steer you towards a thriving, balanced life.

Recognizing that each person is a unique entity with distinct needs is crucial. What proves effective for one may yield different results for another. As the landscape of health and wellness undergoes continuous transformation, a pivotal tool to master is monitoring your progress. This practice is indispensable for attaining long-term health and well-being objectives. By meticulously tracking your journey, you equip yourself with unique data emphasizing the value of tracking progress and understanding one's needs. This data will offer profound insights into understanding your body better. Your body is a powerful means to tune in to the signals it sends, providing vital information on nurturing and supporting it.

Furthermore, the overarching goal of this book is to not only enhance your immediate well-being but to fortify your defenses against potential chronic illnesses. It is a commitment to preventive health measures designed to empower you with the knowledge and strategies to safeguard your long-term health. By implementing these insights into your daily life, you're taking proactive steps towards building a resilient and robust foundation for the years ahead for a healthier, resilient, harmonious connection within you and your environment; all interconnected with the universal symphony of all that is.

This book is my contribution towards propelling humanity forward as a healthier, more vibrant version of themselves, fortified by the guidance of a higher power/God/Universe/Supreme being (or whatever belief system resonates with you). It offers wisdom grounded in the belief that with knowledge and conscientious action, we can forge a path to optimal health, vitality, and a profound sense of well-being toward a thriving, balanced life.

With immense gratitude, I extend my heartfelt thanks to my beloved family, dear friends, and esteemed colleagues. It is through your consistent support and encouragement that this journey has become a reality. Special thanks to Glennis Medina for always being there to listen to my crazy ideas and for creating the 21st-day meal challenge for this book. Special thanks to the Garden of Neuro for helping me deliver this baby! (Yes! You read that right), this book is my baby. Our collective experiences shape a more vibrant version of ourselves.

To you, dear reader, I express my most profound appreciation. Your presence reading this book shows your commitment to wellness and self-discovery. Congratulations on taking this important step. Embrace every challenge on your health journey, never give up, and keep trying to be healthier. Celebrate every action, no matter how small. Thank you, dear one, for being part of this incredible journey.

Before I start introducing you to this book, I want to tell you three things:

1. Get a pen or pencil.
2. This book will ask you some reflection questions as you go. Try not to skip them. These reflecting questions are vital for your journey towards a healthier you. So, you can apply your knowledge and transform it into wisdom immediately.
3. A story on how I got into my health and wellness journey.

"Health is not valued till sickness comes."
Thomas Fuller.

Introduction

Hola. I'm Solanyi Ulloa, proud to be a full-time Mom, Nurse Consultant, Transformational Coach/Speaker/Author. Why mention these titles? Well, they're not just letters; they represent the hard work and dedication I put into earning them to help myself and be able to help you. They symbolize my passion for personal growth and my insatiable thirst for knowledge, even in subjects that some might consider dull. So, while many may think they know me, they might be in for a surprise reading this book!

Getting on board the health train wasn't a smooth ride for me. It all began in 2012 when I found myself in the emergency room with excruciating pain in my back, just below the ribcage on both sides. The pain was sharp, relentless, and seemed to radiate to every corner of my body. It was a level of discomfort that surpassed even the intensity of birthing a 10-pound baby without pain relief – yes, those can be excruciating. My fatigue was debilitating, but I attributed it to chronic sleep deprivation. For nearly a year, I only got 2 to 3 hours of sleep each night. The constant nausea was another challenge, and I can assure you pregnancy was not the cause. I thought it was the cheap food options I used to select daily at the college campus, where I had most of my meals. After several tests, the doctor returned with an almost mischievous smile, asking, "Good news or bad news first?"

The bad news? So, being the hot-blooded Latina I used to be, I rolled my eyes and answered: "Tell me the bad news first." He proceeded: "Well, young lady, your kidneys are shutting down, and you are going into kidney failure." My mind was racing, and I could only picture my poor baby without a mother and me missing her significant milestones.

At that time, she was less than one year old; I was

enjoying motherhood despite all the challenges as a single full-time mom, full-time student, and having a full-time job without family around and less than three friends that I trusted. I cannot tell you how many thoughts I had in milliseconds. Everything in the room was spinning so fast. As a nurse, I knew what that meant. I started to hyperventilate, and my mind raced, worrying about who would take care of my baby if I died. I started sweating and going into a full-blown active panic attack. All I could say was: "Wait, what????"

He explained that the good news was they had identified the issue. Then the doctor said, "The good news is your kidney failure is reversible; we will get you more IV fluids, and you will be good to go, BUT if you do not take care of yourself, I'm afraid your kidneys will end up shutting down. Just keep hydrated, and you will be fine." So, he walked away without giving me information on how to make habit changes to remain hydrated. I could not ask any questions because I had lost my voice, and I was very insecure about my heavy Hispanic accent at the time, not to mention I was still in shock.

It was a wake-up call about the state of my health. The diagnosis was a result of a combination of factors, including chronic stress, poor diet, and a lifestyle that paid little attention to self-care. It was a turning point that forced me to reevaluate my priorities and how I was showing up for myself. This experience began my transformative journey towards a more balanced life. It wasn't just about alleviating the immediate symptoms and embracing a holistic health approach encompassing physical, mental, and emotional well-being. This journey has ups and downs, but it has ultimately led me to a place of profound gratitude for the human body's resilience and the power we hold to shape our health destiny.

Before that pivotal visit to the emergency room, my daily hydration routine followed a predictable pattern. Mornings, I started with a large cup of coffee, a ritual that seemed as essential as the sunrise. By the time 10 a.m. rolled around, the second cup of coffee was already in hand, fueling my efforts on the bustling college campus. Lunch came with a choice between a 20-ounce Pepsi or a 20-ounce Coke, setting the tone for the afternoon. At

2 p.m., it was another 20 ounces of cola, a midday pick-me-up. By 4 p.m., a small glass of water made a fleeting appearance, overshadowed by the looming presence of more coffee or soda. Evening hours, from 8 to 10 p.m., saw a continuation of this caffeine-powered marathon, a bid to stay alert and focused for late-night study sessions.

Yet, amid this demanding routine, a chapter added a unique layer of challenge. Like clockwork, around 2 or 3 a.m., my little one would stir, breaking the stillness of the night. In those tender hours, I'd find myself cradling her in one arm, swaying gently and weaving lullabies into the quiet darkness, coaxing her back to slumber. With my free hand, I'd dive into my studies, determined to forge ahead. Each time I eased her back into her bed, there was a flicker of hope for uninterrupted rest, only to have it dashed as she stirred again. This nightly ritual, a dance of maternal love and academic pursuit, became the backbone of my existence.

Then, on one transformative night, a decision emerged from exhaustion and determination. I chose to continue my studies with my daughter in my left arm, a fusion of maternal duty and scholarly endeavor. In that shared space, we forged a bond that transcended the boundaries of conventional routines, an emblem of the resilience born from sacrifice and the commitment to a brighter future. This singular act would become a touchstone for the journey that lay ahead.

Through trial and error, I initially believed that I would achieve proper hydration by incorporating an additional 2-3 glasses of water each day. However, I soon discovered this was different. The culprit lay in my continued consumption of caffeine, a diuretic that effectively takes water from the body. Despite my efforts, which included persistently drinking 3-4 cups of coffee daily, the water I consumed failed to replenish my body's vital hydration. So, I decided to start on a journey of self-education, determined to unlock the secrets of hydration. My quest bordered on obsession, with each day bringing new revelations. I immersed myself in seminars, workshops, and extensive literature reviews. Health fairs became a trove of insights, and I conducted clandestine experiments to pursue solutions for my unique physiology.

Armed with this new knowledge, I extended my teachings to patients, family, and friends, eager to share the transformative potential of a well-hydrated life. Yet, I understood that change can be a formidable challenge, and only some were ready to embrace it. I respected their autonomy, continuing to offer guidance regardless of their readiness to implement lifestyle shifts.

One fateful evening in 2019, I returned home after an arduous day. My last patient visit had taken me to a home so overwhelmed by clutter that every step was a delicate dance to avoid collision. The air was tainted with a toxic blend of human decay, and insect infestations lurked in every corner. This patient, a non-compliant diabetic, found solace in the persistent haze of cigarette smoke that filled the confined space. His struggles extended beyond the immediate, manifested in an ostomy (surgical opening to divert bowel movements to the abdomen) with an elusive seal, a testament to the challenges he faced. In this distressing case, the patient's condition was exacerbated by an infected Foley catheter, a medical device designed to assist in urinary drainage. Regrettably, the infection led to a severe complication where the penile area experienced a distressing purulent discharge, indicative of the significant level of discomfort and medical urgency the patient was facing. The constant pulling of the Foley catheter caused his penis to split in half. This situation highlights the critical importance of proper medical care and interventions in cases where such complications arise, underlining the need for timely and effective treatment.

The litany of ailments seemed endless: diabetes, congestive heart failure, peripheral vascular disease, chronic obstructive pulmonary disease, and the list went on. This patient's body bore the scars of this relentless battle, with wounds that bore witness to the severity of his condition. Stage 3 and 4 ulcers, proof of the ravages of time and neglect, marked his arms, legs, and coccyx. His skin, once a protection barrier, now echoed the texture of decay. Reptilian scales were a delightful beauty when compared to this patient's skin.

In this somber setting, I forged ahead, offering countless sessions of education and empowerment, hoping to ignite a spark of change. However, the patient's choice remained rooted in the familiar despite the gravity of his circumstances. His story, though just one among many, is a poignant reminder of the profound impact of choice on health and well-being.

It takes tremendous strength and compassion to confront such complex realities. I became a transformational coach to help those who want to create awareness, prevent diseases, and manage existing illnesses to avoid complications. I constantly continued witnessing the tragic consequences of poor lifestyle choices:

- New onset of Diseases.
- Disease complications.
- Alive Human Decomposition.
- Death

The primary focus in nursing school and medical education has traditionally been treating diseases. While this is undoubtedly crucial, there has been a historical gap in the emphasis on prevention. This gap is critical, as preventing diseases improves individual health outcomes and lessens the burden on healthcare systems and society.

Over the years, there has been a growing recognition of the importance of preventive healthcare. Efforts are integrating comprehensive education on prevention strategies into medical training. This shift acknowledges that promoting health and well-being is as significant as treating ailments.

As you start or continue this path, you are at the forefront of this evolving paradigm. You embody the proactive spirit needed to shift the healthcare landscape towards a more holistic, preventive approach. You are taking a stand for a future where individuals receive empowerment with the tools and information needed to lead healthier, happier lives. Your commitment to prevention proves your dedication to your health. By seeking knowledge and resources to prevent diseases, you enhance your well-being and position yourself as an advocate for a healthier society.

7 Strategies to Optimize Your Health & Prevent Chronic Illnesses.

In my journey to better health, I have witnessed the profound impact that lifestyle modifications can have on individuals. It's a remarkable experience to see people regain their vitality and rediscover a sense of purpose and joy. An incredible potential lies within each of us to shape our health outcomes. It's a journey that has allowed me to connect with people on a deeply personal level, walking alongside them as they navigate the path to optimal health. This journey is about more than personal growth; it's about being part of a transformative movement in healthcare.

One case particularly close to my heart is a client with about 15 chronic illnesses. Her multiple diseases seemed to compete. Her heart, lungs, and kidneys locked in a race to see which would give out first. But throughout our coaching sessions, she managed her conditions. Her specialists couldn't believe the improvement in her kidney laboratory test results. She managed to reverse stage 4 kidney disease to stage 3 and maintained it steadily for over a year. She listened attentively and took action steps, discovering what worked best for her unique body. She effectively managed her diabetes, saw improvement in her skin issues, and kept her lung issues from further deterioration. She was determined to have a healthier life; she was optimistic and ready to continue her healthy journey. Later, a malignant stage 4 tumor was found on her right lung, a consequence of over 20 years of excessive smoking. She was determined to fight for her life, but in the end, cancer won the battle. Still, I must say her last days were filled with joy, laughter, and love despite the agony of her pronounced breathless cough, leading her to max out on oxygen usage and continuously increase her medications. Despite her increased efforts to live a healthier life, the damage to her body was irreversible. Hence, I urge you to initiate your health now.

The decision to embark on the health journey stems from a profound understanding of the critical need for preventative healthcare. It goes beyond the conventional model of treating illnesses as they arise. Instead, it's about proactively empowering individuals to make informed choices about their health. It's about breaking down barriers, dispelling misconceptions, and providing a roadmap for those eager to take control of their health narrative. Furthermore, being a health and life coach is more than just a profession for me; it's a true calling fueled by a profound passion for the well-being of every individual I have the honor to coach. One invaluable lesson I've learned in this journey is that it's not about drastic overnight changes but the consistent effort and small, sustainable adjustments that accumulate over time. It's about understanding that every individual's path to wellness is unique, and what works for one person may not work for another. This insight has been a guiding principle in my approach to coaching and developing strategies to meet diverse needs. This endeavor is deeply personal. It signifies a commitment to perpetual learning, keeping pace with the latest wellness advancements, and refining strategies that better guide and support individuals on their unique health journeys. It's a path marked by growth, compassion, and empowerment, and I am wholeheartedly dedicated to seeing it through.

Through this journey, I've witnessed the remarkable resilience of the human spirit. Seeing individuals overcome seemingly insurmountable challenges with determination and grace is inspiring. This resilience reinforces the belief that with the proper support, guidance, and resources, we all can transform our lives. Moreover, I've come to appreciate the profound impact of mindset on our health journeys. Cultivating a positive outlook and a sense of self-compassion can be transformative. It's about acknowledging that setbacks are part of the process and that each day is an opportunity for progress, no matter how small.

My passion for education and empowerment has only deepened. I've seen firsthand how knowledge can be a catalyst for change. It's not just about providing information but about empowering individuals to take ownership of their health, to ask questions, and to make informed decisions. I'm also continually reminded of the importance of community and support networks in our wellness journeys. Sharing experiences, challenges, and triumphs creates a sense of belonging and fosters a supportive environment for growth.

Self-reflection holds an undeniable power throughout all of this. It's about tuning in to your body, listening to what it tells you, and responding with kindness and care. This self-awareness is essential to a meaningful and sustainable health journey. So, as you continue this endeavor, do so with a deep sense of purpose and a profound belief in the potential for positive change. It's about more than just health; it's about a holistic transformation encompassing mind, body, and spirit. And I'm grateful for the opportunity to share this journey with you.

What inspires you to be a healthier version of yourself?

_____
_____
_____
_____
_____
_____
_____
_____
_____
_____

The question I get asked the most is: How do I keep myself motivated on my health and wellness journey?

I remind myself daily of my goals and the deliberate steps I'll take to achieve them. It's a practice that roots me in purpose and propels me forward. Simultaneously, I hold fast to the understanding that no one on this earth is inherently superior to me, just as I am no better than anyone else. This recognition cultivates a deep sense of humility and a profound connection to humanity. In this journey, I have discovered an abiding joy that emanates from aligning with my life's true purpose. It's a joy that permeates even the most challenging moments, as a steady compass that guides me through life's setbacks and flow.

Furthermore, I embrace patience as a steadfast companion. It's a quality that allows for self-compassion, acknowledging that growth takes time and every step forward, no matter how small, is a triumph. Through this, I have forged an unbreakable bond with myself, rooted in love and acceptance, regardless of circumstances or perceived shortcomings. Perhaps most importantly, I have honed the art of energy allocation. Instead of expending valuable resources dwelling on problems, I redirect that energy toward productive problem-solving. It's a transformative shift in focus, one that has paved the way for breakthroughs and empowered me to overcome challenges with resilience and grace.

As I reflect on this journey, I'm reminded that it's not just about reaching the destination, but about savoring each step of the path. It's about embracing the full spectrum of human experience—the triumphs, the setbacks, and everything in between. This journey attests to the limitless potential residing within every individual, waiting to be unlocked with intention, self-love, and a resolute commitment to growth.

What are things you do or can do to keep yourself motivated on this health & wellness journey?

My pursuit of a healthier self is rooted in the desire for a harmonious union of body, mind, and soul. It acknowledges that true well-being transcends physical health alone; it encompasses mental clarity, emotional equilibrium, and a profound sense of purpose. This interconnectedness forms the solid foundation of a life with intention, authenticity, and fulfillment.

It's the aspiration for a life where daily medications and their potential side effects do not hold sway over my quality of life. Instead, I envision a life brimming with boundless joy, where I can engage in any activity that calls to me, unrestricted by health concerns. This vision extends to cherished moments with my daughter, niece, and nephews. I yearn to partake in their journeys, embracing each experience with vigor and presence. Whether it's a playful romp in the park or a quiet moment of shared reflection, I want to be fully present and actively engaged. In nurturing this holistic balance, I find myself not merely existing, but truly thriving. It's a state of being where every facet of my being aligns with its intended purpose. It's an invitation to savor each moment, to relish the richness of experience, and to dive deep into the boundless potential that resides within us all. This vision is not merely a destination; it's an ongoing journey, a commitment to honor the gift of life with vitality, purpose, and presence.

What inspired you to be a healthier version of yourself? Be as detailed as possible.

_____
_____
_____
_____
_____
_____
_____
_____
_____
_____

What chronic illnesses run in your family? (Grandparents, parents, siblings, aunties/uncles, and or cousins).

_____

_____

_____

_____

Why do you want to have a healthier way of living?

_____

_____

_____

_____

This book is a valuable resource to guide readers through a comprehensive spectrum of essential concepts, from foundational to advanced levels. The intention is to empower individuals with the requisite knowledge, whether initiating a health journey for the first time or seeking to deepen their understanding and commitment. The focus is creating a seamless integration of mind and body, recognizing the connection between mental and physical well-being. For beginners, it is a comprehensive initiation, offering insights into the fundamental principles of a holistic approach to health. For those already on the path, the advanced concepts allow them to refine and expand their knowledge to continue making an informed commitment to facilitate a united and balanced approach to health where mental and physical aspects are seen not in isolation but as interconnected components.

Body awareness is a foundational lesson in this transformative journey. Cultivating a clear understanding of your body's needs involves:

- Interpreting its signals.
- Discerning its unique requirements for optimal functioning.
- Paying attention to decode its cravings.

This awareness is instrumental in adopting an individualized approach, where the ability to recognize what harmoniously aligns with your unique body becomes a catalyst for transformation. This insight empowers you to nurture your body to find its full potential. In nutrition, a strategic selection of foods that complement your specific goals and aspirations to shape a dietary regimen that not only fuels your body but also supports your objectives. Furthermore, achieving digestive harmony is crucial, as understanding the foods that positively resonate with your digestive system provides valuable insights, laying the groundwork for a harmonious relationship with your digestive processes.

This journey invites you to explore your body and the nourishment it receives. It's an opportunity to create a deep connection with your physicality, nurturing it with the care and wisdom it deserves. By the end of this exploration, you will possess a wealth of knowledge and a profound understanding of how your inner universe operates.

Get ready for this transformative health journey. First and foremost, I want to express my gratitude for your presence here. Your commitment to educating yourself about making healthier choices is a decisive step towards empowerment for yourself and your loved ones. This book is a labor of love, written with dedication and care, and I'm thrilled to share it with you. You will find the journey of reading it as enriching as my experience in writing it.

Within these pages, you'll gain access to insights that have taken me and countless other years to accumulate. However, it's important to remember that this knowledge, while valuable, is only as powerful as the actions you take based on it. Please follow through with the action steps outlined in each lesson. By doing so, you will take deliberate, manageable steps toward implementing lasting lifestyle changes that will significantly enhance your overall health.

It's not about dwelling on where you've been or even where you stand today; it's about envisioning where you aspire to be. Consistency will serve as your compass in your journey towards wellness. Consider the time you spend engrossed in this book as sacred "Me Time." Establish clear boundaries around this time, recognizing that life's demands may occasionally intervene. In those moments, you'll develop the discernment to prioritize based on the immediacy of the situation.

With dedication and commitment, this journey promises to be a catalyst for positive, lasting change in your life. Throughout our time together, I will provide you with some recommendations so you can take action steps to achieve your wellness goals. We will work one step at a time and sometimes stack new behaviors with pre-existing ones so you can transition smoothly to a healthier lifestyle and have a long-lasting transformation.

I know in this present age and time, we do not want to wait or go step by step, and unfortunately, many people have failed because they want to run before, they learn to walk, but I get it, and believe me, this has been me too. There are diets out there; you name them, and I will probably have tried them at some point, and you probably have tried them too.

I will guide you each step of the way. Please learn from my clients, patients, family, friends, and even the mistakes I have made in my health journey, which I will describe here. But, if you are the type of individual who likes to learn from their mistakes, go for it. I believe in saving time and energy and learning from those who have already made mistakes.

Just remember, you will get what you put in, meaning your effort and willingness to follow the action steps will determine your success with this book and lifestyle choices, but the healthier version of yourself you are creating.

Disclaimer: It's crucial to emphasize that this book is not a substitute for professional medical advice. Its purpose is to offer information and insights on optimizing the health journey. Please consult with your primary healthcare provider before starting a new health regimen. Your PCP (primary care provider) has the expertise and knowledge of your medical history, conditions, and requirements, enabling them to offer advice and guidance.

7 Strategies to Optimize Your Health & Prevent Chronic Illnesses.

This book provides recommendations for informational purposes only. Everyone's health needs are unique, and what works well for one person may not be suitable for another. Your primary healthcare provider is your best resource for understanding how the information in this book aligns with your personal health goals and circumstances. Their insights will ensure that your actions are in harmony with your health profile. Your health is a precious and individualized journey; seeking professional advice is a fundamental step towards optimizing your health journey.

Pivoting Moments: There will be days when you effortlessly adhere to every recommendation, feeling accomplished and on track. Other days may present challenges, tempting you to revert to old habits. But halt; it's crucial to understand that forming new habits is a process that requires time and persistence. Don't be disheartened by momentary setbacks. Instead, view them as pivotal moments—a chance to acknowledge the stumble, regain your equilibrium, and continue your journey toward the healthiest self. Life throws unexpected circumstances our way, yet we try to maintain a sense of hope and positivity. Regardless of what unfolds, make it a priority to finish reading this book and put into practice the wisdom you acquire. On days when discouragement looms large, discipline will stand as your steadfast ally.

By the conclusion of this book, you should be able to:

- Say goodbye to the anxiety of restrictive diets.
- Let go of apprehensions surrounding dietary choices.
- Release self-criticism for occasional slip-ups.
- Embrace the empowerment of intuitive eating, savoring meals that nourish your beautiful body.
- Strategically adjust your habits to harmonize with the healthier version of yourself.

Every step you take is progress. Trust the journey, and above all, trust yourself.

Healthcipline

Let me introduce you to a revolutionary concept I coined "**Healthcipline**." It's an approach to making healthier choices that feels intuitive and organic. It hinges on a simple yet profound principle: tuning into what your body needs, not necessarily what it craves. It's about rationalizing the benefits of the food before you, aligning it with the vision of a healthier you. One crucial aspect is the language we use with ourselves and others. For instance, when faced with a food item on the more nutritional spectrum, like fruits or vegetables, stating that you don't like it can inadvertently shape your perception. Take my own experience as an example. There was a time when I avoided vegetables, opting for an extra portion of meat instead. I vividly recall my reluctance when faced with a bland, boiled broccoli. The mere thought of it was enough to trigger a distasteful reaction.

Yet, fast forward to today, and my perspective has drastically shifted. Before I consume vegetables, I contemplate the wealth of nutrients they'll impart to my body. This shift in mindset has been transformative. The power of our thoughts and words shapes our relationship with food. By reframing our perceptions, we open the door of appreciation for the nourishing potential of every meal. With gratitude, I acknowledge nature's provision of this nourishment that supports my body and mind. Rather than reverting to transient diets that often result in deprivation and malnourishment, I choose the path of sustained healthier choices.

It's not about forcing yourself to like something, but rather, allowing yourself to rediscover it in a new light. Your journey to a healthier you begin with these small, conscious shifts in perspective. This more profound exploration of health discipline is the language of our relationship with food. It also emphasizes the potential for transformation through a change in mindset. The essence of health discipline lies in the cultivation of enduring, healthful routines. This is a commitment to carry with you throughout your life's journey, a pledge to prioritize and nurture your body in the most natural and beneficial ways possible.

If you find yourself harboring negative associations with healthy foods, it's an opportunity for healing and release. Thank the memory or emotion for its presence, and then gracefully let it go. Recognize that the benefits far outweigh any perceived risks or lingering negative thoughts. Sometimes, this process may necessitate repeated reinforcement until it becomes second nature. Persistence is key.

Consider me your allied guide in this transformation toward your healthiest self. I'm eager to witness your progress. Believe in yourself, for you are entirely capable of achieving this! Your journey is marked by growth, empowerment, and a flourishing state of well-being.

Journaling Time

What are your thoughts on Healthcipline?

_____
_____
_____
_____
_____
_____
_____
_____
_____
_____
_____
_____
_____
_____
_____

"Prevention is better than cure."
English proverb.

Chapter 1

Disease Prevention Road Map

Many chronic illnesses share a typical underlying pattern in terms of their disease progression. This pattern often involves gradually building up risk factors or triggers, including small genetic predispositions, lifestyle choices, environmental exposures, and other contributing factors. As these factors accumulate, they can lead to subtle changes at the cellular or molecular level within the body. These initial changes may not manifest noticeable symptoms but set the stage for developing more significant health issues.

As time passes, the body's natural regulatory mechanisms may struggle to maintain balance due to these accumulating risk factors. This imbalance can lead to a tipping point where symptoms become apparent; after a thorough examination, the healthcare provider puts together all the puzzle pieces and comes up with a diagnosis that accurately reflects the patient's health status. From this point onward, the disease typically follows a progressive course, often involving periods of exacerbation and remission. Without effective intervention or management, the condition may continue to worsen, potentially leading to complications or co-morbidities.

Understanding this typical pattern is crucial for healthcare professionals in developing effective prevention and treatment strategies. Identifying and addressing the early stages of this disease's progression may make it possible to intervene before the condition advances to a more severe or irreversible state; this underscores the importance of proactive lifestyle modifications and targeted interventions in managing chronic illnesses. However, disease prevention encompasses comprehensive strategies aimed at averting the development or progression of illnesses. This proactive approach is grounded in the understanding that many chronic conditions share common risk factors, and by addressing these factors early on, we can significantly reduce the likelihood of disease emergence.

Prevention begins with creating health awareness and education from reliable sources. It empowers individuals with the knowledge and tools to make informed lifestyle decisions; this includes promoting balanced hydration, a healthy mind, balanced nutrition, regular physical activity, avoiding harmful habits like smoking or excessive alcohol consumption, and healthy boundaries. Furthermore, it extends to environmental factors, advocating for clean air, water, and safe living conditions.

Screening and early detection programs play a vital role in prevention. They allow healthcare providers to identify risk factors or early signs of diseases before they progress to a more advanced stage. Regular check-ups and screenings are particularly effective in conditions like cancer, cardiovascular disease, and diabetes, where early intervention can be transformative.

Embracing a holistic approach also encompasses mental health. Promoting mental well-being, stress reduction, and access to mental healthcare services are fundamental aspects of preventing conditions like depression and anxiety disorders.

Importantly, disease prevention is not solely an individual responsibility but a collective effort involving healthcare providers, policymakers, communities, and society. It calls for policies supporting healthy living, ensuring access to quality water, quality foods, and less harmful chemicals, and creating environments conducive to overall health. Ultimately, disease prevention is a dynamic and multifaceted endeavor that promises to improve individual health, reduce the burden on healthcare systems, and enhance the overall quality of life for communities worldwide.

Imagine your inner universe as this incredibly complex and fascinating organism. It is not just a solo act confined within your body; it is a dynamic system that collaborates and interacts not only with itself but also with the environment and the vastness beyond. Each component plays a unique role, contributing to the harmonious balance.

Health On Demand Nurturing the Universe Within

Have you ever experienced the beautiful and mesmerizing dance of life? We all participate in a thrilling and unpredictable performance, each with unique moves and rhythms. From the highs to the lows, every step we take contributes to this incredible dance, making it an adventure worth savoring.

Every tiny cell in your body is amazing—it is alive and conscious and works with its buddies to keep you going. These cells are not loners; they are all part of a team, and the way each one does its thing adds up to the extraordinary, orchestrated symphony of life inside you. Think of it like a community where each member plays a crucial role. So, every cell is not just doing its own thing but contributing to the organism as a whole and keeps you ticking.

Think about it—just like your fingerprints set you apart from everyone else, your voice and heartbeat are also one-of-a-kind. Your voice carries its distinct melody and your heartbeat, well, it is like your personal rhythmic signature. No one else sounds or beats quite like you. It is part of what makes you unique, well, you! You have your built-in tune, complete with its own beat, frequency, vibration, and energy field, making it all extraordinary. Your voice and heartbeat add their special notes to the grand, majestic, and universal composition. Think of it like this: You are not just walking around with a heartbeat and a voice; you have your own personal soundtrack. Your heartbeat is not just a thump-thump; it is a rhythmic signature that's unique to you. Just as each snowflake in nature boasts its individual pattern, and no two sunsets paint the sky the same way, your voice and heartbeat contribute to the unique melody of the human experience. Similarly, no two human beings share identical rhythms.

Furthermore, here is the real magic—your tune is not just playing for you; it is part of a grand orchestrated symphony that includes every living thing. It is like your personal rhythm is a note in a song that connects with nature's beat, other living organisms, and universal energy. So, in every thump and word, you contribute to a musical masterpiece beyond just you— the extraordinary harmony of existence. So, ensure your contributions to the collective are positive and uplifting. Your unique tune has the power to inspire, resonate, and create a ripple effect of goodness in the lives of others.

3

In choosing positivity, you enhance your own melody and contribute harmoniously to the collective tune that plays across the interconnected web of existence. It is the beautiful dance of individual notes coming together to create a song that elevates the spirit and brings joy to the universal melody. So, let your tune be a light of positivity into the larger composition of life's extraordinary existence.

Imagine your human design and creation as a canvas, and you are like a special thread in the big, beautiful quilt of life. Each thread is different, just like you are. Your uniqueness adds cool colors and patterns; other living organisms and the universe co-create this colorful masterpiece with you. It is like being part of a team where everyone has a unique role to make something awesome. It is like you are a crucial piece in a giant puzzle, making the whole picture more exciting and complete.

The connections extend beyond the body's physical boundaries, creating a web of interdependence with the world around us. Our inner universe is not just a standalone entity; it is a vibrant, interconnected ecosystem where every part influences and is influenced by the more extraordinary cosmic dance of existence. Embracing this perspective adds a profound layer of understanding to the complexity and beauty of the inner universe.

Prevalent patterns underline the development of numerous chronic diseases. These complex processes are at the core of our cellular functioning, shedding light on critical factors such as mitochondrial dysfunction, autophagy, glycation, oxidative stress, insulin resistance, membrane instability, inflammation, and methylation (Lusting, 2021).

Mitochondrial dysfunction

What are Mitochondria? The mitochondria are responsible for converting food into energy. The cell uses this energy to do all its activities, such as moving, growing, and repairing itself. Another way to think about mitochondria is as the batteries of the cell. They store energy so the cell can use it when needed. Imagine that your body is a car. Your mitochondria are the engine of your vehicle. They burn food to create energy, which powers your car. Without mitochondria, your body would not be able to function. You would not be able to move, grow, or even think. Mitochondria, often termed the "powerhouses" of our cells, play a crucial role in energy production, breaking down nutrients like glucose and fatty acids (the relationship between fat and the food we eat) to fuel various cellular functions.

Unhealthy foods often contain abundant processed components, unhealthy fats, and excess sugar. These constituents can potentially harm the functioning of mitochondria, resulting in a condition known as mitochondrial dysfunction. This state disrupts various bodily functions, leading to symptoms like fatigue, muscle weakness, cognitive fog, and difficulty concentrating.

A common feature in various chronic diseases is mitochondrial dysfunction. These conditions encompass a wide range of ailments, including neurodegenerative disorders like Alzheimer's, Parkinson's, Huntington's disease (progressive brain disease), Amyotrophic Lateral Sclerosis, best known as ALS (affects the brain and spinal cord causing nervous system and musculoskeletal system failure), and Friedreich's ataxia (a rare genetic progressive disease that causes the affected person neurological and physical impairments), as well as cardiovascular issues such as atherosclerosis and other heart-related conditions. Additionally, it plays a role in diabetes, metabolic syndrome, autoimmune diseases like multiple sclerosis, lupus, and type 1 and Type 2 diabetes, neurobehavioral and psychiatric disorders like autism, schizophrenia, and mood disorders, gastrointestinal problems, fatiguing illnesses such as chronic fatigue syndrome and Gulf War illnesses, musculoskeletal conditions including fibromyalgia and muscle hypertrophy/atrophy, various forms of cancer, and chronic infections.

Autophagy

Autophagy is the body's recycling system at the cellular level. It enables the body to break down and repurpose old or damaged cell components, enhancing the efficiency of cell operations and generating fresh energy sources, thus playing a vital role in preserving cell well-being and preventing diseases.

Within each cell lies a multitude of components essential for its functioning. Over time, some parts may become faulty or cease functioning, becoming discarded or superfluous material within an otherwise healthy cell.

Autophagy serves as the body's means of recycling and rejuvenating cellular components. It empowers a body cell to break down its superfluous elements, salvaging the usable fragments to construct new, functional cell parts. This process allows cells to discard what they no longer require. Moreover, autophagy acts as a quality control of the body cells. When a cell accumulates an excess of unnecessary components, it can impede proper functioning. Autophagy transforms this disorder into the specific, vital cell elements needed for optimizing body cells for overall performance.

Fasting stands out as one of the most potent triggers of autophagy. During fasting, the body depletes its glycogen reserves and utilizes fat for energy, prompting the activation of autophagy. This process aids in the removal of damaged cells.

Foods with processed ingredients containing unhealthy fats, added sugar, excessive salt, and detrimental trans and saturated fats, can provoke inflammation and cell damage and hinder autophagy. Fast food, in contrast, typically contains an abundance of processed ingredients, unhealthy fats, and added sugar. These components can provoke inflammation and harm cells, thereby hindering autophagy and giving rise to various health issues.

Glycation

All right, imagine your body as a giant puzzle. Sometimes, sugar molecules, like tiny puzzle pieces, stick to proteins and fats inside your body. This puzzle-sticking process happens faster when we eat foods that are not very healthy, like ones with lots of processed things like extra sugar and not-so-good fats.

This process makes something called "advanced glycation end products," or AGEs. Think of them like little troublemakers. They can cause problems within blood vessels, nerves, and organs. It is like when too many stickers cover a page, and you cannot see what is underneath.

These troublemakers can lead to serious health issues like diabetes, heart problems, Alzheimer's, and even cancer. So, we must be careful about how much sugary and unhealthy food we eat. We want to keep those troublemakers at bay and our bodies as healthy as possible!

Oxidative Stress

Our bodies engage in various essential processes, from digestion to metabolizing substances introduced to the body like alcohol and prescribed drugs, all of which produce harmful compounds known as free radicals. Typically, our natural antioxidant system works to neutralize these. However, if this system falters, it can set off a chain reaction that harms cellular processes, hinders cell division, damages DNA, and impairs energy production.

Oxidative stress stimulates immune responses and triggers allergic diseases, such as asthma, allergic rhinitis, atopic dermatitis, and food allergies; this indicates that patients with allergic diseases have an outdated antioxidant protection system compared to healthy individuals (Sackesen et al., 2008). Antioxidant supplementation could compensate for increased inflammation and oxidative stress in asthma patients. However, excessive supplementation can heighten susceptibility to allergic diseases and asthma (Murr et al., 2005).

7 Strategies to Optimize Your Health & Prevent Chronic Illnesses.

The modern lifestyle, characterized by an unhealthy diet, lack of physical activity, and exposure to various chemicals, can contribute to oxidative stress; this, in turn, contributes to the rising burden of chronic diseases, as supported by numerous studies (Fenga et al., 2017; Docea et al., 2018; Fountoucidou et al., 2019; Kostoff et al., 2020). This comprehensive review provides robust evidence that antioxidants may play a role in alleviating certain chronic-degenerative conditions, as well as promoting healthy aging.

Storytime: The Battle of the Body Machine

Once upon a time, in a land not too far away, there was a marvelous machine that did incredible things. The Body Machine was responsible for turning food into energy, healing cuts, and even keeping away pesky germs.

Nevertheless, deep inside this machine were tiny troublemakers called free radicals. They loved causing mischief and sometimes made the Body Machine work not as smoothly as it should. Luckily, there were also superheroes known as antioxidants. They were like the guardians of the Body Machine, swooping in to catch the troublemaking free radicals.

One day, the Body Machine got tired, and the troublemaking free radicals started to outnumber the antioxidants; this made the machine a bit wonky. Some parts did not work as well, like a puzzle missing a few pieces. It was like when a computer screen flickers because something inside is not quite right. Some cells were not doing their jobs, and the instruction manual, known as DNA, got a little smudged. It was like the Body Machine spoke a language only a few understood.

As time went on, the troublemakers began to create even more problems. The Body Machine did not feel good; it was like a brave knight fighting a dragon with a rusty sword. The land was in danger of falling into darkness.

However, then, a wise healer arrived and shared a secret. "Eat colorful fruits and vegetables," the healer said, "and take care of the Body Machine. That way, more superheroes will come to help, and the troublemakers will not stand a chance!"

The people of the land listened, and they started to fill their plates with vibrant foods. The antioxidants grew more robust and more numerous, ready to fight off the troublemakers. The Body Machine began to hum with energy and vitality once more.

With the superheroes by their side, the Body Machine defeated the troublemakers and restored balance to the land. The cells worked harmoniously, and the instruction manual, DNA, was once again clear and crisp.

From that day on, the people of the land understood the importance of caring for their Body Machine. They knew that some help could do amazing things and keep them healthy and strong for years to come, as they all lived happily and healthily ever after. The end!

Insulin Resistance

Imagine your body like a car. Eating food, especially things like bread, rice, or pasta, turns into a kind of sugar called glucose. This glucose is like the fuel for your car. Your body has a unique part called the pancreas that makes insulin. Insulin is the key that helps the glucose get inside your cells to give them energy. It is like the key that starts your car. However, sometimes, especially if you overeat sugary or eat processed foods a lot, your body cells can start to ignore the insulin. It is as if your car's lock stops working, and the key no longer opens the door. So, even though you have a lot of glucose (or fuel) in your body, your cells cannot use it correctly; this is called insulin resistance. It is like having too much fuel but not being able to put it in your car's tank, making you feel tired and not as strong as you should be. Eating healthy foods like fruits, vegetables, and whole grains is essential to keep your body's insulin working correctly, just like ensuring your car's key and lock are working right!

Membrane Instability

Let us imagine our body cells are like little houses with solid walls around them. These walls are called the "cell membrane." They are like the fences around houses that keep everything safe and sound.

However, sometimes, these cell membranes get weak. When that happens, we call it "cell membrane instability." It is like when a fence around a house is not as strong as it should be. When the cell membrane is unstable, it can lead to some problems. It is as if the walls of a house started to wobble; this can cause things inside the cell to not work correctly. Unhealthy foods, like those with lots of processed stuff, unhealthy fats, and too much sugar, can worsen this problem. These foods can be bullies to the cell walls. They can weaken them and make them more likely to have problems.

Moreover, if the cell walls are not solid and steady, it can lead to serious health issues, like parts of the cell not working or even the cell not surviving. It is a bit as if a house's walls got so weak that the whole house could not stay up properly. So, eating healthy foods is vital to keep our cell walls strong and our bodies healthy! That way, everything can work as it should, and we can stay happy and strong.

Inflammation

Inflammation is a natural response when our body is injured or fighting an infection. Short-term inflammation, like when we get a cut, the skin swells, turns red, and hurts; this usually goes away in a few hours.

Inflammation may induce a sensation of heat, impede function, or present with inconspicuous symptoms. If it does not go away and becomes chronic, it could lead to more tissue damage and disease. Chronic inflammation can last for months or even years and is linked to over half of global deaths. Studies have shown that our environment can play a role in inflammation, which is connected to various diseases like autoimmune conditions (like rheumatoid arthritis), heart problems, digestive disorders (like Crohn's disease), lung diseases (like asthma), mental health conditions (like depression), diabetes, neurodegenerative diseases (like Parkinson's), and certain cancers.

Exposure to chemicals, germs, or radiation can cause tissue inflammation. Inflammation is the body's natural response to injury, infection, or harmful substances. The body says, "Hey, something is wrong; let's fix it!" Usually, this is a good thing and helps us heal. However, eating a lot of fast food, which often contains processed ingredients, unhealthy fats, and added sugar, can lead to chronic inflammation; this is when the inflammation sticks around for a long time, which is not good.

The problem with chronic inflammation is that it can harm the body cells and tissues over time. It is like a small fire that keeps burning and contributes to serious health issues like heart disease, diabetes, and even some types of cancer. So, to keep our bodies healthy and happy, it is a good idea to ingest minimal fast food and focus more on eating nutritious foods like fruits, vegetables, whole grains, and lean proteins. This way, we can help reduce the risk of chronic inflammation and keep our bodies running smoothly.

Methylation

Methylation is like a tiny worker in our bodies that helps with essential tasks. It involves things like repairing our DNA and controlling how our genes work. It is crucial for keeping our bodies running smoothly. Now, when we constantly eat unhealthy foods, it can affect this little worker, methylation. It is like giving the worker some tools that are not quite right for the job.

Overeating unhealthy food can sometimes make methylation work less effectively and lead to problems in how our genes function, which can contribute to health issues like heart disease, diabetes, and even certain types of cancer. Reduced methylation leads to a drop in dopamine production. This change in dopamine levels affects the balance of other neurotransmitters. Consequently, individuals may experience difficulty focusing, concentrating, short-term memory, organization, emotional stability, healthy sleep patterns, and hormone regulation. So, focusing more on eating nutritious foods like fruits, vegetables, whole grains, and lean proteins is a good idea. This way, we can help support our little workers and methylation, and give our bodies the proper tools to keep us as healthy as possible and to prevent chronic illnesses.

Programmed Cell Death Apoptosis

Apoptosis, often called "programmed cell death," is a crucial process in the human body that plays a fundamental role in maintaining balance, eliminating damaged or potentially harmful cells, and ensuring proper development and functioning of various biological systems. Apoptosis is a highly regulated and controlled cellular process. It is essential for average tissue and organ growth, development, and maintenance. Most body cells have a ticking clock; when the body cells do not follow this pattern, they go rogue, known as cancer cells.

Initiation of Apoptosis: Various internal and external signals can initiate apoptosis. These signals can include genetic instructions:

- Cellular stress.
- DNA damage.
- External factors like hormone levels, toxins, or immune responses.

Apoptosis regulates a complex network of signaling pathways within the cell. These pathways involve a series of molecular events that lead to the activation of specific proteins, known as caspases, which play a central role in executing the process of apoptosis. Apoptosis has several distinct phases:

Initiation: This phase involves the activation of specific signals or receptors that trigger the apoptotic pathway.

Execution: Once initiated, a series of biochemical events occur, activating caspases. Caspases destroy cellular components, including DNA fragmentation, protein degradation, and membrane alterations.

Cleanup: After dismantling cellular components, the cell undergoes changes that enable it to undergo phagocytosis. Neighboring cells or specialized immune cells, which means dedicated body cells, will eat up the parts of the dead cells, preventing the release of potentially harmful cellular contents.

Physiological Roles of Apoptosis

Tissue Homeostasis: Throughout life, apoptosis helps maintain tissue balance by regulating the number of cells in various tissues and organs. It removes damaged or dysfunctional cells, preventing the accumulation of potentially harmful cells.

Immune System Function: Apoptosis regulates the immune response. It eliminates immune cells after an infection, preventing excessive inflammation and tissue damage.

Preventing Cancer: Apoptosis is a protective mechanism by eliminating cells with DNA damage or mutations, reducing the risk of uncontrolled cell growth and tumor formation.

Embryonic Development: Apoptosis is crucial in shaping the developing embryo by sculpting tissues and organs, eliminating no longer-needed structures.

Implications of Apoptosis for Health and Disease: Dysregulation of apoptosis can have significant implications for health and disease. Insufficient apoptosis may contribute to cancer and autoimmune diseases, while excessive apoptosis can lead to neurodegenerative disorders, tissue atrophy, and degenerative conditions.

Therapeutic Applications: Understanding apoptosis has led to the development of targeted therapies for conditions like cancer. Drugs that modulate apoptotic pathways are used in cancer treatment to induce cell death in cancerous cells.

7 Strategies to Optimize Your Health & Prevent Chronic Illnesses.

Our unhealthy dietary choices disrupt apoptosis and the gut microbiome; these choices can be imprinted in our genes, impacting us and future generations. While our modern diet addresses nutrient deficiencies, the surplus of calories and specific macronutrients can lead to heightened inflammation, reduced infection control, elevated cancer risks, and greater susceptibility to allergies and auto-inflammatory diseases. The Western diet, characterized by excessive saturated and omega-6 fatty acids, inadequate omega-3 fats, excessive salt, and refined sugar, is well-known for its detrimental effects on the heart, kidneys, and overall body weight. However, it is increasingly evident that this diet also affects our immune system. This impact furthers various aspects of modern living, including reduced exposure to microorganisms, increased pollution, elevated stress levels, and numerous other well-documented factors.

In summary, apoptosis is an essential biological process that maintains tissue health, contributes to development, and safeguards against cellular abnormalities. Its understanding has far-reaching implications in fields ranging from basic cellular biology to medical interventions and therapies. The human body is so unique that it regularly passes inventory and is "this cell is sick, kill it, remove it from the body, and create a new healthy cell that can carry the important function."

Unlocking the Secrets of the Body's Building Blocks: A Journey into the World of Cells

The human body has an army of cells that defend it from external and internal threats, the "immune system." For the array of cellular functions to work harmoniously, they require the proper nutrition and hydration to keep the body as healthy as possible.

"Cells Rely on Proper Nutrition for Optimal Functioning."

Cells are the basic building blocks of the human body, and they perform various essential functions to keep you alive and healthy. These functions include:

Energy Production: Think of your body as a highly efficient power plant. It converts the food you eat into a type of fuel called glucose. Your cells then use this glucose to generate the energy needed for all activities, from essential functions like breathing and digesting to more strenuous activities like running or lifting weights. Your pancreas is the central control for energy consumption and metabolism. Findings of a study on autopsy tissues published in the European Journal of Endocrinology published in 2020 showed that the outer cells of the pancreas that help with digestion undergo significant changes and degradation over time. Poor diet and poor hydration =cell chaos leads to disease.

Waste Elimination: The body is like a self-cleaning machine; it has an incredible way of removing waste through various systems. The digestive system eliminates solid waste through bowel movements, the skin removes waste via sweat, and the respiratory system removes waste with each breath. After using nutrients for energy, the metabolic processes produce waste products.

Did you know that your kidneys are vital to keeping you healthy? They work hard to filter out waste products from your blood, which are then excreted as urine. Pretty impressive, right?

Tissue Repair and Growth: The body is in a constant state of renewal. Cells are continuously dying and replaced, which is particularly important for tissues that undergo a lot of wear and tear, like skin, blood cells, and the lining of your digestive tract. Proper nutrition and hydration are crucial for this process.

Immune System Function: Your immune system is a complex network of cells, tissues, and organs working together to protect your body from harmful invaders like bacteria, viruses, and fungi. Proper nutrition supports the immune system by providing the nutrients it needs to function optimally.

Hormone Regulation: Hormones are chemical messengers that help regulate various bodily functions. For instance, insulin helps regulate blood sugar levels, while thyroid hormones regulate metabolism. Nutrients from your diet play a key role in producing and regulating these hormones.

Nervous System Communication: Your nervous system relies on a complex interplay of chemicals and electrical signals to transmit messages between your brain and the rest of your body. Adequate nutrition and hydration are crucial for maintaining the health and function of nerve cells.

Muscle Contraction: Muscles are responsible for all forms of movement, from walking to blinking. Muscle contractions require various nutrients, including calcium, potassium, and magnesium. Dehydration or nutrient deficiencies can lead to muscle weakness and cramps.

Blood Clotting: When you get a cut or injury, your body must quickly stop the bleeding; this relies on a complex process called blood clotting. Nutrients like vitamin K heavily influence this process.

DNA Synthesis and Repair: Your DNA contains the instructions for every process in your body. Proper nutrition provides the building blocks needed for DNA replication and repair, ensuring the healthy functioning of your cells.

Oxygen Transport: Hemoglobin, a protein in your red blood cells, binds with oxygen in your lungs and carries it to every cell in your body. This process is vital for cellular respiration, where oxygen is used to produce energy.

Digestion and Nutrient Absorption: Your digestive system breaks down food into essential components like carbohydrates, proteins, and fats. These nutrients are then absorbed into your bloodstream and distributed to cells for various functions. According to a group of Swedish researchers led by Dr. Frisén, the cells that form the gut lining are notably one of the shortest-lived cell types in the entire body, with a lifespan of only five days. However, it reveals an intriguing perspective: studies in mice have shown a stomach cell lining lifespan of three to five days. Since mice and human gut lining have similarities, excluding these swiftly regenerating cells, the average body should be able to regenerate more cells to protect the stomach lining from disease-causing agents. When you consistently consume highly processed foods, sugary foods, and sugary beverages, along with other not-so-nutritious options, your body may not be able to generate high-quality cells that can protect the lining of your stomach, leading to potential health issues down the road.

Temperature Regulation: Your body maintains a stable internal temperature, regardless of external conditions crucial for optimal enzyme function and metabolic processes. Thermoreceptor cells work by trying to provide balance. For example, you sweat to cool down; you shiver to generate heat when you are too cold.

Fluid Balance: Water is involved in nearly every bodily function. It helps regulate body temperature, aids digestion, and acts as a medium for chemical reactions. Proper hydration is crucial for maintaining this delicate balance. Kidney cells work in conjunction with intestinal cells, blood cells, lung cells, skin cells, and many other cells to maintain proper nutrition and hydration to work optimally.

Neurotransmitter Production: Neurotransmitters are chemicals that transmit signals in your brain. They play a crucial role in mood, behavior, and cognitive functions—nutrients like amino acids, vitamins, and minerals needed for their synthesis. Brain cells work effortlessly to exchange information and ensure optimal body functioning. Memory and cognitive function require proper nutrition to support brain health, influencing cognitive function, memory, and learning. Nutrients like omega-3 fatty acids, antioxidants, and vitamins and minerals are crucial to brain function.

Detoxification: Your liver is the primary organ responsible for detoxifying harmful substances from your body. It transforms toxins into less harmful compounds that can be excreted. This process relies on various cells to transport nutrients, including antioxidants. Hepatocyte (liver cells) lifespan can range from 200 to 300 days, but of course, many factors influence this lifespan.

Bone Health and Density: Calcium, vitamin D, and other minerals are essential for maintaining strong and healthy bones. Your bones can become brittle and prone to fractures without proper nutrition and hydration.

Vision and Eye Health: Nutrients like vitamin A, lutein, and zeaxanthin are crucial for maintaining good vision and preventing eye conditions. They help protect your eyes from oxidative damage and support overall eye health. Proper nutrition and hydration help the body eliminate dead cells and create new ones to keep the organs working properly and prevent illnesses.

Inflammatory Response: Inflammation is the body's natural process to respond to injury or infection. However, chronic inflammation can lead to various health issues. Proper nutrition and hydration, particularly anti-inflammatory foods, can help regulate this response. Your immune system cells are constantly patrolling the body for foreign invaders.

Hormone Regulation and Endocrine Health: Hormones influence various bodily functions, from metabolism to mood. Proper nutrition is essential for producing, regulating, and balancing hormones.

Mental Health and Well-being: Nutrition and hydration play a significant role in mental health. A balanced diet with the proper nutrients and adequate water intake can help regulate mood, reduce the risk of mental health disorders, and support overall health.

pH Balance: The body carefully regulates its pH levels, maintaining a slightly alkaline environment. Please note that a too-alkaline or too-acidic pH is not optimal. Adequate nutrition and proper hydration help maintain this balance, crucial for enzyme function, cell health, and many other bodily processes. Your body carefully regulates its pH levels, keeping it within a range for enzyme function, cell health, and many other bodily processes.

Diets high in processed foods, meat, dairy, and sugary drinks can cause the body to become acidic. When the body is too acidic, it can lead to several health problems, including kidney stones, muscle cramps, osteoporosis, gout, headaches, arthritis, fatigue, and skin problems.

A diet high in fruits, vegetables, and whole grains helps to balance the body's pH levels by balancing alkalinity and acidity, creating a suitable environment for cells to thrive and function optimally.

It is important to note that the effects of diet on the body's pH levels remain a field of study. Some research suggests that diet has a minimal effect on blood pH, while others suggest that diet has a more significant effect on the pH of other bodily fluids, such as urine. More research is needed to determine the full impact of diet on the body's pH levels and overall health. However, eating a balanced diet high in fruits, vegetables, and whole grains is an excellent way to overall health.

Regarding nutrients, we refer to the essential elements our body needs, such as vitamins, minerals, proteins, carbohydrates, fats, and water. These nutrients play crucial roles in cellular metabolism and cellular growth.

For example, proteins are essential for the structure and function of cells. They are involved in processes like enzyme production, immune response, and cell signaling to ensure each cell does what it needs to do. Carbohydrates are the primary energy source for cells, especially for high-energy-demanding tissues like the brain and muscles. Cells require a steady supply of nutrients to carry out these tasks efficiently. Vitamins and minerals act as cofactors in various biochemical reactions. They help enzymes perform their functions effectively. Without these micronutrients, many cellular processes would slow down or even halt.

Water, the most critical nutrient, is involved in nearly every cellular function. It serves as a medium for chemical reactions, helps regulate temperature, and assists in transporting nutrients and waste products within the body. Now, imagine depriving your cells of these essential nutrients. It is like asking them to work without the proper tools and materials. They would struggle, and their performance would suffer, leading to a range of health issues, from fatigue and reduced cognitive function to weakened immunity and impaired tissue repair.

Without proper food and hydration for an extended period, your body cells may be compromised; they may not have the necessary resources to function optimally, leading to a significant drop in overall performance.

Eating processed food is like going without food because the cells do not get the proper nutrition to perform the various tasks they need to achieve. Providing your body with a balanced and nutritious diet should be a non-negotiable endeavor to ensure that your cells receive the nutrients they need to carry out their vital functions effectively.

The rule of thumb is to get all these nutrients naturally if possible. If you use supplements, select an organic and reputable brand since many supplements are poorly regulated and contain more harsh chemicals that will cause harm instead of benefits. Taking multiple supplements simultaneously is not beneficial since each supplement can cancel out the benefits of the other supplement.

Rule of thumb for selecting supplements:

Ideally, talk to a health care professional to get laboratory tests done to determine deficiencies, and based on the results, work on a supplement plan.

- Select a supplement brand with high-quality ingredients, such as many organic ingredients.
- Select supplements with a minimal chemical ingredient list free of added chemical dyes.
- Supplement brand that is third-party tested to ensure safety and that the list of ingredients is what is in the product.
- Avoid deceptive claims. Supplement claims must be realistic. Many marketers and supplements will claim the product's ability to treat severe health conditions.

"To enjoy good health, to bring true happiness to your family, to bring peace to all, first discipline and control your mind."
Buddha.

Chapter 2

MINDSET

Learning Objectives:

- Setting Yourself Up for Success
- Gratitude on the Daily "GOD"
- Clear the clutter!
- Managing Negative Thoughts
- Nurturing Positive Thoughts
- 5 Minutes Morning Routine
- 5 Minutes Night Routine
- Boundaries

A mindset is a set of beliefs about oneself and the world that influences how one thinks, feels, and behaves. It is a filter through which we see the world and ourselves. There are two main types of known mindsets: fixed and growth.

A fixed mindset is the belief that our abilities are fixed and cannot be changed. People with a fixed mindset believe they are either smart or not intelligent, talented, or not talented, and so on. They believe their intelligence and abilities result from genetics or other factors beyond their control. People with a fixed mindset are more likely to give up easily when faced with challenges. They may also be more likely to attribute their successes to luck or external factors and their failures to internal factors, such as their lack of intelligence or talent.

A growth mindset is the belief that our abilities can be developed and improved through hard work and effort. People with a growth mindset believe they can learn new things and improve their skills, no matter how old they are. They believe intelligence and abilities are not fixed but can be developed through hard work and dedication. People with a growth mindset are more likely to persevere and overcome challenges. They are also more likely to attribute their successes to their hard work, effort, and failures to factors they can control, such as a lack of preparation or a bad strategy.

Mindset is vital because it can significantly impact our success in life. People with a fixed mindset are more likely to give up easily and avoid challenges, while people with a growth mindset are more likely to persevere and achieve their goals.

There are several things that we can do to develop a growth mindset, such as:

Challenge yourself regularly. Challenging yourself regularly is one of the best ways to develop a growth mindset; this could mean taking on new challenges at work or school, learning a new skill, or trying something you have never done before. Challenging ourselves, succeeding, and recognizing that hard work and effort can develop our abilities, revealing that they are not fixed.

Celebrate successes, no matter how small. Celebrating your successes is essential, no matter how small; this helps build your confidence and self-esteem, which is essential for developing a growth mindset.

Learn from past mistakes. We all make mistakes, but it is important to learn from them. When you make a mistake, try to understand why it happened so you can avoid making the same mistake in the future.

Set challenging goals. Setting challenges forces you to stretch and learn new things, which is a great way to develop a growth mindset.

Be open to feedback. Feedback can be a great way to learn and grow. When you receive feedback, be open to it and see it as an opportunity to improve.

Be patient. Developing a growth mindset takes time and effort. Do not expect to change overnight. Just keep challenging yourself learning from mistakes, and being open to feedback, and you will eventually develop a growth mindset.

Find a mentor. A mentor can be a great help in developing a growth mindset. They can provide guidance, support, and encouragement.

Read books and articles about growth mindset. There are many excellent books and articles about growth mindset. Reading about it can help you understand it better and how to apply it to your own life.

Talk to people who have a growth mindset. Talking to people who have a growth mindset can be inspiring and motivating. They can share their stories and experiences and help you see that developing a growth mindset is possible.

Believe in yourself. Believing in your ability to learn and grow is the most important thing. If you believe in yourself, you are more likely to take risks, challenge yourself, and learn from your mistakes.

In conclusion, mindset can significantly impact our success in life. We must develop a growth mindset to achieve our goals and believe that we can learn and grow. Mindset impacts thinking, emotions, and behaviors. Mindset can be fixed, or it can grow. A fixed mindset cannot be changed; people with a fixed mindset tend to give up easily and avoid challenging activities. A growth mindset allows individuals to develop new abilities and skills, learn from mistakes, take on new challenges, embrace setbacks, and move on. Individuals with a growth mindset tend not to give up easily; they see challenges as growth opportunities and replace negative thoughts with positive ones.

Setting Yourself Up for Success: Approaching this healthy journey with a positive and determined mindset can positively influence your success. A positive attitude will lead to a positive outcome: "I can do this" and "I got this," you are setting yourself up for accomplishment. This mindset means you believe in yourself and your ability to achieve your goals. Even if you do not believe in yourself fully, start practicing and believing it. Create a mental toolkit with self-confidence, motivation, and an "I can do it" attitude. This tool kit will be a priceless asset on your path toward the healthiest version of you. With this positive outlook, you are more likely to learn valuable information and take empowered action in your daily life.

Each small step towards better health is in the right direction away from illness. So, keep that positive attitude close and watch how it helps turn your aspirations into reality. Your belief in yourself is a powerful force that can push you forward on this journey. Embrace it and trust in your ability to succeed.

What is your main goal for reading this book?

_____

_____

_____

_____

_____

When do you want to achieve this goal?

_____

_____

_____

_____

_____

When will you know that you have achieved your goal?

_____

_____

_____

_____

How will you keep yourself motivated throughout this health journey?

_____

_____

_____
_____
_____

What are three obstacles that may come in the way of you completing reading this book?

_____
_____
_____
_____
_____

What are three solutions you can implement to prevent the above obstacles?

_____
_____
_____
_____

"Who has health has hope, who has hope has everything."
Arab Proverb.

Daily Gratitude: As you wake up to a new day, take a few moments to reflect on all the things that you are grateful for in your life. It could be your good health, the love and support of your family and friends, the comfort of your home, or the satisfaction of your job. Allow yourself to bask in the warmth of these positive thoughts and start your day on a thankful note.

As soon as I wake up, I make it a point to take a deep breath and express my gratitude for the gift of life. One great way to cultivate a positive mindset is to keep a gratitude journal. It is a simple but powerful activity involving writing down things you are thankful for. You can choose to write down a few things each day, or you can take some time once a week to reflect on what you appreciate in your life. By consciously focusing on the good things, you can train your brain to notice and appreciate the positive aspects of your life, leading to increased feelings of happiness and contentment. Over time, you can reflect on your journal entries and see how your gratitude has evolved and grown, providing even more motivation to continue this rewarding practice. I have two gratitude journals. I keep one by my nightstand, and the smaller one I carry with me when traveling occupies less space, and the weight is less.

Practice mindfulness: Mindfulness is paying attention to the present moment without judgment and focusing on good things in your life.

My favorite mindfulness practice is taking a few deep breaths throughout the day and checking my emotions to see if anything that happened that day could be draining my energy.

Spend time with loved ones: Spending time with loved ones is a great way to feel grateful for the people in your life. Try to connect with loved ones who lift you and nurture your energy, those who take out the best version of yourself, try to connect with them regularly, whether it is going out for coffee, taking a walk together, or just spending time talking via video call or voice call. On the other hand, it is okay to love from a distance the individuals that weigh you down or drain your energy.

Being Kind to Others: Helping others without expecting anything in return. If someone needs help and you can help, great. Also, volunteering your time within institutions that align with your values is an excellent way to help others. Charity donations and helping estrangers whenever you can.

Take Time to Celebrate: When you celebrate the small things in life, you will be happier, more positive, and more connected to the world around you by simply being a happier version of yourself.

We all have encoded contagious emotions that trigger learning responses in our DNA to help us survive. Let us use this smartly and allow the positive emotions to make us feel fulfilled.

Storytime: Sandy's Transformational Gratitude Journey

In a world consumed by external and internal noise, meet Sandy, a human under stress, unmet expectations, and relentless deadlines. Her life was a race against time, leaving her drained and unfulfilled.

One day, she started a daily gratitude ritual that soon reshaped her world. She started by writing down three daily blessings, and her perspective shifted. She focused not on scarcity but on life's abundance—the warmth of the morning sun and the laughter of loved ones—all took on new meaning.

This gratitude practice became her daily ritual, planting seeds of positivity in her soul. With each passing day, those seeds flourished, bathing her heart in radiance. Her mood improved, stress became more manageable, and contentment enveloped within her.

Sandy's gratitude did not stop at her journal. She shared her appreciation, strengthening bonds and creating a kinder, harmonious relationship with those around her. Life's challenges still arose, but Sandy faced them with the gratitude forged shield.

Her journey of thankfulness radiated outward, inspiring others to start on their gratitude journeys. Grateful hearts multiplied, making the world a better place. Sandy's frantic race against time had transformed into a purposeful journey of appreciation and fulfillment. Gratitude, her guiding light, revealed beauty in adversity and unveiled profound richness in life.

Sandy's story illustrates that gratitude is a transformative journey. It shifts perspectives, enhances well-being, strengthens bonds, and gracefully empowers us to face life's challenges. Amidst life's chaos, gratitude reminds us that even in darkness, there is always something to be thankful for. The end!

Clearing the clutter is essential for a multitude of reasons:

- It enhances mental clarity by creating an organized environment that nurtures clear thinking and effective decision-making.
- It reduces stress, providing a more peaceful atmosphere that nurtures productivity.
- A clutter-free space promotes creativity and allows for better focus on tasks.

Beyond the mental benefits, decluttering contributes to better physical health by reducing allergens and improving air quality. It also positively impacts emotional well-being, instilling a sense of control and order. Living or working areas feel more extensive and comfortable with more space available. Furthermore, a clutter-free environment can strengthen relationships by minimizing stress and tension. Lastly, it encourages mindfulness about possessions, prompting consideration of their value and purpose. Clearing clutter creates an organized, harmonious, and peaceful space, enhancing one's quality of life on multiple levels.

Start small. If you are the type of person who gets overwhelmed by large tasks, start with one area or room. Do not try to declutter the entire home in one day; it will only make you more likely to give up.

Set a timer. Give yourself time to declutter, such as 30 minutes or an hour, to help you stay focused and tell your mind you can get a lot done in that time frame.

Plan. Before you start decluttering, take a few minutes to plan to stay organized and find out what area you want to declutter first, second, third, and so forth.

Get rid of things you do not use or need. If you last used something in the past year, it is time to eliminate it from your space. You can donate it to a local charity, or garage sale, or sell it online. Set up a time frame by when you will get rid of that; if donating it, set a date and time to drop it off; if you sell it, set a date and time for when the items need to be gone by.

Get help from a friend or family member. Having someone to help you can be a great way to stay motivated and get it done faster.

Listening to music or podcasts while decluttering can help you stay focused and make the time go by faster.

Take breaks. Do not try to declutter for hours on end. Take breaks every 20-30 minutes to stretch, walk around, or get a snack.

Reward yourself. When you finish decluttering a room or area, it may feel empty or weird at first, reward yourself with the freedom and great view of a decluttered space, which, from my point of view, helps with mind decluttering.

Managing Negative Thoughts

The brain has approximately 100 billion neurons (brain cells). These cells are intertwined by trillions of synapses (neuron connections). These connections are constantly transmitting and exchanging information. The human brain functions like a computer, sending and receiving chemical and electrical information from the body's cells, the senses, and surroundings. The brain is the processing center for all bodily functions, emotions, and decision-making. The brain operates on a picture-like approach, like in a movie film. When we see something, the brain initially receives the input upside down. Within milliseconds, this information is relayed to the occipital lobe (back of the head) for processing. This visuospatial information is decoded, including factors like depth perception, color determinants, distance, object, and face recognition, thus creating memories, meaning, and emotions associated with the environment.

The way the brain stores memories for future use is comparable to a library shelf. It receives information, stores it on a mental shelf, and retrieves it when needed. However, in cases of poor memory or cognitive impairment, such as those with dementia and traumatic brain injuries, this retrieval process may be challenging. Throughout our lifespan, the brain's size and weight change.

The average adult female brain weighs 2.7 pounds, while the adult male brain weighs 3 pounds (sorry, guys □, science is science, and data is data). The brain is the organ that demands the most energy, requiring approximately 20% of daily energy due to the multitude of managerial tasks it performs. This energy demand may increase during tasks that require higher cognitive demands. The human brain operates 24 hours a day, 365 days a year, to sustain life. Its composition includes approximately 60% fat and 40% water, salts, protein, and carbohydrates. The water composition in the brain can be as high as 80% when considering hydrostatic and osmotic pressure. Hydrostatic pressure refers to fluid volume, while osmotic pressure involves the balance of water in and out of cells. Studies have shown that the brain areas supporting emotions, social interactions, and cognitive functions remain adaptable to change, thanks to the creation of new learning opportunities through neuroplasticity.

Have you ever wondered what shapes your thoughts and actions? Well, let me tell you about the mind. According to psychoanalyst Sigmund Freud, our way of thinking encompasses conscious, preconscious, and unconscious thoughts. Conscious thinking occurs when we are actively aware of our thoughts.

The preconscious is a powerful force made of beliefs, ideas, and memories that has a massive impact on our daily lives. It is unconscious but easily accessible when needed to be recalled (forming part of long-term memory). Unconscious thoughts tend to be automatic and often influence our behaviors. These unconscious thoughts significantly shape how we perceive ourselves, others, and the world around us.

A thought is a construct created from opinions, beliefs, emotions, ideas, sounds, and images, shaping our creative perception of the world. These mental constructs often emerge as automatic responses, whether real or imaginary. It is theorized that a single thought comprises an astounding 1,000 neurochemical signals per second.

Individuals often seek external solutions, turning to family, friends, and acquaintances for advice. While brainstorming can be a valuable exercise, it is imperative to recognize that the answers we often seek reside within us.

The challenge lies in accessing this internal wisdom, particularly when we struggle to discern our inner voice's true intentions and purpose; this can be attributed to the constant demands of our busy lives, the pervasive noise in our environments, or, in more challenging cases, the presence of unresolved trauma waiting to seize any moment of quiet reflection.

The encouraging news is that one can overcome these barriers by cultivating mental discipline. Doing so gives you the power to cultivate a resilient state of psychological well-being. Consider disciplining the mind, like attending a school or gymnasium for the mind. You can assert control over your thoughts through deliberate efforts, ensuring they serve you constructively rather than allowing them to dictate your experiences and reactions.

Managing Negative Thoughts (MNT)

Negative thoughts can significantly impact your well-being, often leading to feelings of stress, sadness, and a sense of being stuck. It is important to understand that completely suppressing or controlling these thoughts can be challenging, as they are a natural part of the human experience, arising as a means of self-preservation.

Human minds have evolved to shield us from inherent human tendencies like greed, ignorance, and hatred. These deeply ingrained patterns have been passed down through generations via genetic coding information, contributing to our identities. This genetic interplay may explain why specific thoughts and behaviors do not always align with the true divine self or the individual you aspire to be. Recognizing this dynamic relationship is a crucial step toward personal growth. By cultivating an awareness of thoughts that no longer serve your best interests, you gain the ability to regulate your mental landscape. This mindfulness allows you to examine emerging thoughts and discern whether they align with your desires and aspirations. Through this process, we take charge of our narrative and follow a more positive transformational journey towards self-discovery.

7 Strategies to Optimize Your Health & Prevent Chronic Illnesses.

Let me introduce a method I labeled LAF. This helped me become aware of my mind and thought patterns and unite my mind and body.

LAF Method

Label:
- Recognize it as a thought product of your mind. Thoughts are mental constructs that may or may not align with objective truth.
- Thoughts are influenced by your perceptions, emotions, and past experiences.
- Understanding that a thought is not an absolute representation of reality allows you to maintain a balanced perspective.

Acknowledge:
- Acknowledge the thought and explore its origins without judgment.
- Where is this thought coming from?
- What triggers it? Is it a specific situation? or an experience? Or your current emotional state?
- Do you have evidence to support the thought? Once you have examined the evidence, explore alternative perspectives.
- Is this thought based on actual circumstances? Or is it a product of subjective interpretation? Examine the evidence and explore alternative perspectives.

Flip:
- Is this a new or recurrent thought?
- If it is a recurrent thought, why has it surfaced?
- Is this thought influenced by your surroundings?
- If the thought had a voice, what would the voice try to tell you? Or if it had a color, what would that color be?

- Thank the thought once you have figured out what is trying to tell you. Then, move on to the present moment and transform that negative thought into a new positive one. Ask yourself if there are other ways to view the situation that may be more balanced or constructive. This process of cognitive reframing can lead to a more accurate and empowering interpretation. You might consider instances where you've successfully tackled challenging projects, demonstrating your capability, this evidence can counteract the negative thought.

By following these steps, you engage in a process of introspection and critical thinking. This empowers you to not only understand your thoughts but also to actively shape them in a way that aligns with your goals, values, and true capabilities. It's a powerful tool for promoting positive self-talk and a healthier mindset.

Common negative thoughts and cognitive distortions:

Extremism: seeing situations as perfect or a complete failure without considering the middle ground. "All-or-Nothing Thinking."

Drawing sweeping conclusions from one negative event, assuming it applies to all situations. "Overgeneralization."

Fixating on negatives leads to a skewed perception of reality. "Mental Filter"

Ignoring or dismissing positive experiences reinforces negative beliefs. "Disqualifying the Positive."

Making negative assumptions without solid evidence. "Jumping to Conclusions.

Assuming you know what others are thinking without asking. "Mind Reading."

Believing negative outcomes are inevitable. "Fortune Telling."

Exaggerating or downplaying the importance of events or personal qualities. "Magnification or Minimization."

Assuming feelings reflect reality. "Emotional Reasoning."
Using "should," "must," or "ought to" leads to guilt or resentment. "Should Statements."
Attaching extreme labels based on specific behaviors. "Labeling and Mislabeling."
Taking responsibility for negative events. "Personalization."

Recognizing these patterns helps you in creating healthier thinking and decision-making. By challenging and reframing, distortions can improve your emotional well-being. Acknowledging these cognitive distortions lays the foundation for cultivating healthier thought processes and making more constructive decisions. It is like having a map that guides you toward a more balanced perspective by actively challenging and reframing these distortions, empowering you to see situations more clearly. For example, an "all-or-nothing" thinking mentality, recognizing that there is often a middle ground, allows you to approach challenges differently.

Furthermore, this practice significantly enhances emotional well-being by providing a toolkit to navigate life's ups and downs. When faced with a negative thought, you can apply strategies to shift your perspective, reducing unnecessary stress and anxiety. This process leads to a more resilient and adaptable mindset. You become better equipped to face adversity and navigate complex situations, ultimately contributing to a greater sense of overall well-being. It is a powerful tool that empowers you to control the narrative and lead a more fulfilling life.

Nurturing Positive Thoughts (NPT)

In cultivating a positive mindset, it is vital to direct your focus towards the positive aspects of your life. During challenging moments, a personal mantra I often advocate is to remind oneself, "It could be worse." This simple yet powerful perspective shift prompts gratitude and serves as a potent antidote to negativity. By consciously adopting such affirmations, the spotlight shifts away from adversity, redirecting awareness toward a more nurturing mindset. The practice of gratitude is a luminescent light in the darkest night, setting off a positive chain reaction in your mind. As you infuse your thoughts with positivity, you will observe a transformative shift in your life.

Self-care is an anchor in rebalancing your brain's chemical equilibrium and enhancing your mood. It forms a crucial element in this journey towards positivity. Cultivate a habit of framing situations in a positive light. This positive outlook sets the stage for positive outcomes, ultimately leading to a more positive life. Consider these fundamental practices:

Utilize the LAF Method: Employ the 'LAF' method – Label, Analyze, and Flip – to counteract negative thoughts. This technique, combined with strategies discussed earlier in managing negative thoughts, is potent in reshaping your thinking patterns.

Extend Self-compassion: Extend kindness and patience to yourself on this transformative journey. Recognize that progress takes time, and nurturing positivity is a praiseworthy endeavor.

Mindful Content Consumption: Be discerning about the information you expose yourself to, whether through news, social media, or the company you keep. Opt for content that enriches and uplifts you and aligns with your future self, that self you are in the process of becoming. Refuse anything that does not align with that future version of you.

Surround Yourself with Positivity: Seek out a company that radiates positivity and mindfulness. These influences will serve as pillars of support, particularly when you are tempted to flow back to old behaviors that no longer serve you and no longer align with the future version you are in the process of becoming.

Incorporate Physical Activity: Dedicate at least five minutes each day to physical activity to get started. It is a meaningful step towards enhancing your well-being.

Engage in Joyful Activities: Align your pursuits with the person you aspire to become. Engage in activities that resonate with your most authentic self and bring you genuine joy.

Cultivate Mindfulness: Engage in mindfulness practices to center your mind and find tranquility in the present moment.

Connect with Nature: Immerse yourself in nature or bring its soothing presence through calming sounds, elements, and backgrounds within your environment.

Extend a Helping Hand: Consider ways to contribute to others. Volunteering time with a cause that resonates with you is a fulfilling way to make a positive impact.

Acknowledge Achievements: Celebrate your accomplishments, recognizing their significance, even if they seem minor. Each achievement contributes to your positive journey.

Prioritize Consistency: Understand that transformation is a gradual process. The habits you cultivate should stand the test of time, becoming integral to your lifelong journey of positivity.

Visualize a Positive Future: Envision a future filled with positivity and optimism. This mental imagery serves as a powerful motivator and a guiding light.

Embracing these practices will promote positivity and fortify your mental and emotional well-being. This is a journey of continuous growth, and your dedication to cultivating positivity will undoubtedly yield enduring success.

Storytime: The Melody of Transformation

In a land where shadows dance, and spirits roam,
A tale unfolds of a heart-seeking home.
In minds that harbor storms, both dark and deep,
A symphony of change begins its sweep.

Negative notes, like rain on glass, they fall,
Weighing down the soul, a haunting call.
Yet know, dear heart, that this is but a phase,
For storms must pass, revealing brighter days.

In ancient codes, our nature we inherit,
A collage of traits, both fine and merit.
Yet tangled threads may obscure our sight,
Veiling the path to our inner light.

Greed, ignorance, and hatred's ancient rhyme,
Echo through time, a haunting chime.
Yet within us lies a melody untold,
It is a song of love and kindness, bravery and boldness.

With mindfulness as our guiding star,
We gaze within, both near and far.
Examining thoughts, discerning truth,
If they align with dreams, we hold them in view.

The symphony swells, a crescendo grand,
As we take charge, our destiny is in hand.
No longer bound by shadows of the past,
We rise, transformed, our spirit free at last.

Each note is a step, a leap, a bound,
Through self-discovery, we are found.
Embracing change, we find our way,
In harmonies of night and day.

So let the melody guide your flight,
Through valleys low and mountains' heigh.
For, in the end, the music will reveal,
The truth that sets your spirit free to heal. The end!

5 Minutes Morning Routine

A morning routine can help you decrease anxiety, reduce stress levels, and promote overall physical and mental well-being by setting the tone for a productive and focused day.

- Deep Breathing (1 minute):
- Find a quiet, comfortable spot to sit or stand.
- Close your eyes and take a deep breath through your nose, allowing your lungs to fill.
- Exhale slowly through your mouth, releasing any tension.
- Repeat this deep breathing exercise for one minute; this helps to oxygenate your body, calm your mind, and prepare you for the day ahead. Visualize a positive mindset of the day where your emotional intelligence contributes to mental clarity and cultivates a sense of calm by sending positive and relaxed impulses to your nervous system.
- Gratitude Reflection (1 minute):
- Reflect on three things you are grateful for. They can be simple or significant. It could be the sunshine, a supportive friend, or the opportunity for a new day. This practice sets a positive tone for a grateful mindset.
- Set Intentions for the Day (1 minute):
- You want to accomplish or focus on one or two things for the day. These could be work-related tasks, personal goals, or areas where you want to direct your attention.
- Setting intentions provides a sense of purpose and direction and ensures you continue to work towards meaningful objectives.
- Gentle Stretching (1 minute):
- Stand up and stretch your arms overhead to wake your body up.
- Gently roll your shoulders and neck to release any overnight stiffness.

Stretching improves blood flow, flexibility, and alertness. Hello, new day!

Affirmations (1 minute):

Repeat a positive affirmation or mantra to yourself. Choose an affirmation that resonates with you and reflects the mindset you want to cultivate to reinforce positive thinking and boost confidence by focusing your mind and energy on the good things happening in your life.

Summarizing: This 5-minute routine incorporates deep breathing, gratitude, intention-setting, stretching, and affirmations to promote a positive and focused start to your day. It is easily implementable and can be adjusted to suit your preferences. Consistency is key! You can add more time if your schedule allows. This 5-minute morning routine is realistic, attainable, sustainable, and does not require extensive time. Make it non-negotiable to begin your day with the right mindset, enhance productivity, and establish priorities.

This routine is intentionally designed to integrate seamlessly into your morning, regardless of your schedule. It is flexible and adapts to your lifestyle. On days when time is tight, you can allocate just 1 minute to practice it (no excuses now). On days when you have extra time, feel free to extend stretches or write down more than three things you're grateful for in your gratitude journal.

You can incorporate some of these steps while brushing your teeth, getting dressed, or during any other existing morning routines you may have. The key is to make this a non-negotiable ritual, uniquely adapted to your needs and preferences, to transform each day before it officially begins. Please do yourself a favor: Make it nutritional and as natural as possible when you have something to eat in the morning. I have covered you with breakfast ideas in the nutritional chapter.

5 Minutes Bedtime Routine

A bedtime routine aids the transition, allowing your mind and body to decompress, sending calming impulses to your nervous system, and setting the ambiance for sleep quality. Unplug and Relax (1 minute): Turn off screens and engage in a calming activity like reading one sentence of a preferred book. Avoid TV or electronic devices at least 1 hour before bed, even though researchers suggest it is best to avoid electronic device usage at least 2 hours before bed. Dimming lights is helpful for your internal clock (circadian rhythm).

Reflect on Your Day (1 minute): Take a moment to think about the joyous moments of your day. No matter how small the moment was, celebrate it with all your being!

Express Gratitude (1 minute): Take a moment to think about something you are grateful for. It helps to end the day on a positive note.

Prepare for Tomorrow (1 minute): Lay out what you need for the next day—clothes, keys, or any essentials—this will save time and reduce morning stress.

Mindful breathing (1 minute): Find a quiet, comfortable spot to sit or stand.

- Close your eyes and take a deep breath through your nose, allowing your lungs to fill.
- Exhale slowly through your mouth, releasing any tension.

This routine is designed to seamlessly integrate into your nightly habits, promoting a more relaxed and rejuvenating sleep. As you continue to practice, it will become increasingly effortless. Once you have mastered this 5-minute routine, expand it as your schedule allows.

Boundaries

"Boundaries define us. They define what is me and what is not me. A boundary shows me where I end up, and someone else begins, leading me to a sense of ownership. Knowing what I am and taking responsibility for gives me freedom."- Henry Cloud.

What are boundaries?

Boundaries refer to the limits and guidelines a person establishes for themselves in various aspects of life, including physical, emotional, and interpersonal boundaries. These limits define what is acceptable and comfortable for an individual and protect one's well-being, values, and personal space.

Boundaries can be internal (related to thoughts, feelings, and self-worth) and external (about interactions with others and physical space). They help maintain a healthy balance between giving and receiving, ensuring that one does not overextend oneself or compromise one's needs and values. Setting and respecting boundaries is a crucial aspect of self-care and is essential for maintaining healthy relationships and a positive sense of self.

Setting boundaries is a fundamental pillar of self-care, acting as a shield to safeguard our physical, mental, and emotional health. It is a practice that extends across various spheres of our lives, be it with family, friends, colleagues, or even acquaintances. While it holds immense value, it can indeed be a challenging endeavor. Often, we find ourselves nodding "yes" to the demands and expectations of others, inadvertently neglecting our own needs and desires. It is an inclination deeply rooted in our social fabric, where putting others before ourselves is often lauded. However, it is essential to recognize that establishing boundaries is not selfish or disregard for others; instead, it is a conscious choice to honor the journey.

In a world that's often fast-paced and demanding, boundaries act as a shield, protecting your physical, mental, and emotional health. When you establish boundaries, you communicate your needs, limits, and expectations

41

to yourself and others. This practice is an act of self-respect and self-love. It's a way of honoring your priorities, desires, and values. It grants you the freedom to prioritize self-care without guilt or hesitation. Moreover, setting boundaries is not about being selfish; it is about ensuring you show up as your best self for yourself and those around you. It enables you to conserve your energy for what truly matters, fostering healthier and more fulfilling relationships.

Setting boundaries shows strength, self-awareness, and a firm commitment to your divine self. While it may not always be met with immediate understanding or acceptance, it is a practice that ultimately paves the way for a more fulfilling and authentic existence—so, knowing that you are nurturing yourself and the relationships and connections that genuinely align with your highest self.

Life moves relentlessly, and I once found myself inside a maze of interpersonal relationships, work demands, and personal aspirations. It was like maneuvering through a complex traffic system, each encounter and responsibility a signal directing my path.

Some interactions were like inviting green lights encouraging progress through open communication and mutual respect. These connections felt like a warm embrace where understanding flowed freely. They propelled me forward, infusing my journey with purpose and vitality.

Then came the moments akin to a cautionary yellow light, urging me to slow down and exercise prudence. These were the instances where I learned the art of setting limits on my time and energy. They shielded me from the looming threat of burnout, providing a necessary pause for reflection and self-preservation.

Moreover, there were the red lights, the moments that demanded a firm "stop." These were the boundaries safeguarding my physical and emotional well-being. Recognizing toxic situations and having the courage to step away became essential. These red lights were not a sign of weakness but a testament to my strength and self-awareness.

As I ventured along this path, I encountered resistance from those around me. Labels like "selfish" and "inconsiderate" flung my way. Then, I realized the importance of staying rooted in my vision for personal growth. Like earmuffs against the noise of naysayers, I learned to trust my inner compass.

Setting boundaries was not about isolation but cultivating healthier, more meaningful connections. It was about communicating my needs, respecting the needs of others, and finding a delicate balance. It was an affirmation of my worth, a practice of self-love that allowed me to prioritize my well-being without guilt or hesitation.

Boundaries were not rigid walls but scaffolding, providing structure for personal growth and harmonious living. They guided me through the twists and turns of life, ensuring I moved forward with confidence and grace.

On an airplane, securing your oxygen mask before assisting others ensures your ability to help. Similarly, prioritizing my well-being was not an act of selfishness; it was a prerequisite for being of genuine help to others.

Ultimately, I understood that others' perceptions didn't define me. Deep in my heart, I knew I was not the person they described, and I resisted the urge to prove them wrong. Instead, I channeled that energy into my personal growth, allowing my achievements to speak louder than any words could.

Boundaries in life are like the rules of the road. They guide our interactions, helping us navigate relationships, work, and personal well-being. Imagine them as traffic signals: some boundaries are like green lights, encouraging us to move forward healthily. These include open communication and mutual respect. Like a yellow light, others ask us to slow down and exercise caution. For instance, we are limiting our time and energy to avoid burnout. And then there are the red lights, where we must firmly say "stop" to protect our physical or emotional safety; this could involve recognizing toxic relationships and walking away. As we rely on traffic signals to maintain road order, setting and respecting boundaries creates a harmonious and balanced flow. So, driving, yielding, and stopping when needed is perfectly okay.

In this process, we may encounter resistance from those around us, labeling us as "selfish," "inconsiderate," or even "egotistic." Understanding that such judgments often stem from misunderstanding or misaligning values. Those who might not share your vision for personal advancement may need help to comprehend your choices. It is natural for their perspectives to clash with yours. While this dissonance may initially sting, it is imperative to remain constant in your commitment to personal progress.

Maintaining a genuine focus on your goals and aspirations is a powerful anchor in times of criticism or doubt. It serves as a reminder of the milestones you aim to achieve and the version of yourself you strive to become.

It is like wearing earmuffs against the noise of naysayers, allowing you to stay attuned to your inner compass. Setting boundaries is not an act of closing yourself off from the world; instead, it is a deliberate step toward creating healthier, more meaningful connections. It's about communicating your needs, respecting the needs of others, and creating a harmonious balance.

Boundaries reflect your self-worth and provide the structure needed for personal growth and well-rounded living. So, embrace them as a powerful tool for a more balanced and harmonious life.

When you step onto an airplane, and the cabin prepares for takeoff, you will inevitably hear the flight attendant follow the vital safety instructions. Among them, my favorite now is, "In case of unexpected cabin pressure loss, oxygen masks will drop from above your seat. Please place your oxygen mask on before helping others."

Understanding this concept took me a few years. It was not until I truly grasped the importance of self-care that the message resonated. You see, it's imperative to prioritize your well-being before tending to others. It's akin to securing your oxygen mask before assisting someone else with theirs.

Other people's perceptions of you should not define who you are. Knowing you are not the person they describe, resist the urge to expend your precious energy proving them wrong. Instead, channel that energy into your growth, progress, and endeavors. Let your achievements speak volumes in the silence, for it is in your success that the most resounding noise is made. ☺ .

How to set clear boundaries for success?

If your experience with boundaries is minimal, start small. If you are unsure about the status of your boundaries, no worries – I got you covered. Taking that first step is crucial. Begin by putting pen to paper and writing down your boundaries. Then, step in front of a mirror and rehearse them. Initially, it might feel silly, perhaps even a bit awkward. However, trust me, there is a moment when it all clicks into place, and asserting your boundaries becomes second nature. You will do it without a second thought.

Boundaries are more like the fence around a garden. They keep out the weeds and pests, allowing your vibrant blossoms to flourish. These weeds can manifest as toxic relationships, draining commitments, or even internal self-doubt. By clearly setting and communicating your boundaries, you create a space where your authentic self can grow and thrive.

Think of a ship at sea. Boundaries act as the hull, ensuring it stays afloat even in choppy waters. Without them, the ship would be tossed around, vulnerable to every wave and storm. Similarly, in the sea of life, boundaries provide stability and protection, which is your way of saying, "I value myself, and I deserve to be treated with respect and kindness."

Another way to look at it is to picture it as a shield that guards your inner peace, like a forced field of self-respect and self-worth. It is your way of declaring, "This is how I allow myself to be treated." Boundaries are not about building walls but defining the parameters within which you thrive. They are the foundation of healthy relationships with others and yourself.

 Healthy boundaries are all about finding that sweet spot, the balance between being too permissive and overly rigid. Picture it as walking along a midline, neither veering too far left nor too far right. It is crucial to convey your expectations to others but keep it straightforward. Let them know what is acceptable and unacceptable and be clear about the consequences if those boundaries are not respected.

For instance, I have had to establish boundaries around my time in my journey towards a healthier work-life balance. As someone who is on the path of recovery from workaholism, my family and friends are aware of my busy schedule. If I am engrossed in creating content for my programs or immersed in study sessions, I switch on my 'Do Not Disturb' notifications. If a call does come through, my first response is, "Can I call you back when I am finished here?" This sets the tone that my focused time is crucial. They have come to understand the rhythm of this dance. If they say it is an emergency when it is not, I will politely explain that I will get back to them once I'm done or suggest texting if they need a quicker response.

Being intentional about how I allocate my time has been a game-changer. Those within my inner circle, the ones I have chosen to keep close to understand the importance of my current projects. They respect that my free moments are scarce and valuable. So, when I carve out time for them, it is not about quantity but quality. This shift in approach has allowed for deeper connections and more meaningful interactions.

It is worth noting that setting boundaries is not about shutting people out but about creating a space where you can show up as your best self. It is a way of ensuring that your interactions are fulfilling and mutually respectful. It is about honoring your priorities and, in turn, respecting the priorities of others. As you continue this boundary-setting journey, remember it is a dynamic process. Boundaries may need adjustment as you grow and evolve. Boundaries are a living part of your self-care toolkit, a compass guiding you toward a more balanced and fulfilling life. So, start small, be patient with yourself, and watch as your boundaries become the foundation of a well-lived life.

Achieving a lot in a short time often leads to the question, "How do you manage it all?" My answer remains consistent: boundaries. These boundaries are not just limited to one aspect of life; they extend across various areas of my life, from social media and personal life to professional commitments, business endeavors, leisure activities, and even relationships. Establishing these boundaries has not been a walk in the park, but the journey has been invaluable.

The process of setting boundaries begins with carving out dedicated time. Select a specific day and time, aiming for a slot with minimal potential distractions. If feasible, consider muting your phone and activating the 'Do

Not Disturb' mode. This feature allows for repeated calls in case of a genuine emergency. Communicating this designated time to your inner circle is crucial, emphasizing that you will only be available in an emergency. Let them know that they can call persistently in such cases, ensuring the call will eventually reach you.

Within the confines of your home, especially if others are present, take a few moments to explain that you are engaged in something of great importance - in this case, your health. Stress the significance of this time for your health and well-being. If children are in the household, this is an excellent opportunity to introduce them to healthy habits. Invite kids or your partner to join this health journey with you. It is a chance to work on this path together, reinforcing a sense of unity and shared purpose. Of course, if there are no takers, that is all right. It is better to pursue this endeavor alone than with influences that may not align with your goals.

Consistency is key to create and maintain healthy habits. Stick to a fixed date and time for your lessons and activities. This regularity not only makes remembering your commitments easier but also reinforces the importance of prioritizing them.

To further solidify this routine, set up alarm reminders. Schedule them for 15 minutes before your designated time and then again 5 minutes prior. When the 5-minute alarm sounds, dive into your lessons. This proactive approach keeps you on track and focused. You would be surprised how much can transpire in just a couple of minutes, potentially causing you to lose sight of the commitment you made to yourself.

Boundaries are a powerful tool in letting others know what you are comfortable with and what is not. Consider these examples: You have every right to communicate that unannounced visits are unwelcome. If someone uses a term that does not sit right with you, a simple "I do not welcome that word" suffices. Do not hesitate to ask others to step up and take on more responsibility if you believe it is warranted. The age-old wisdom, "Do not bite off more than you can chew."

Crucially, do not carry guilt for setting boundaries. It is an act of self-love and self-care. You are only obligated to provide lengthy explanations for your boundaries if someone genuinely seeks guidance to respect them or if they are creating their own. While helping others is commendable, sometimes offering advice once and allowing them to make their own decisions is the best approach. If they return with the same issue and have not followed your advice, step back and remind them that you provided guidance. If their situation drains your energy, creating some distance is okay. Your well-being is paramount, and setting boundaries is crucial to safeguarding it.

Setting boundaries can indeed be a demanding task. It requires time and energy but consider this an investment in yourself and your well-being. By establishing boundaries, you're not only demonstrating how you deserve to be treated, but you are also asserting your self-respect. The payoff is immense. It is like reclaiming your energy from an energy vampire draining you. The absence of clear boundaries can lead to burnout, leaving you feeling depleted and overwhelmed.

I highly recommend initiating this practice from day one. Some individuals may embrace it, while others might find it challenging. It is natural to wonder: Do I want someone in my life who does not respect my boundaries? If your answer is a resounding "no," you're on the right track! This decision marks the initial step in the empowering journey of setting and upholding your boundaries. Self-love and self-respect resonate positively in every aspect of your life. You deserve to be surrounded by people who honor and value your boundaries because they are vital for nurturing healthy, fulfilling relationships. So, keep moving forward on this path of self-discovery and growth, knowing you are crafting a life that aligns with your most authentic self.

Boundaries are not rigid or inflexible. They can evolve and adapt as you grow and change. They are a living, breathing part of your self-care toolkit. So, start small, be patient with yourself, and watch as your boundaries become the compass guiding you to a life of greater fulfillment and well-being.

"Lack of boundaries invites lack of respect"- Anonymous.

Questions to ask yourself:

What brings me a sense of fulfillment?

_____

_____

_____

_____

What sparks inspiration within me?

_____

_____

_____

_____

Who are the individuals or groups that recharge me and bring out the best in me?

_____

_____

_____

_____

What situations or aspects leave me feeling dissatisfied? Why do they have this effect on me?

_____

_____

_____

_____

What tends to drain away my inspiration?

_____

_____

_____

_____

Which individuals or groups tend to deplete my energy and bring out the worst in me?

_____

_____

_____

_____

These are the questions I often find myself pondering. Getting started on the journey of setting boundaries was challenging. There were moments of loneliness, but deep down, I knew it was necessary. It meant creating distance, even from close friends and family. It was not an easy decision, especially being someone with high regard for family. The thought of creating that space was initially heartbreaking. Sometimes, I questioned the whole process, wondering if it was worth it. However, a small voice inside me insisted, "You need this distance." I would say, "But it is my family we are talking about!"

The realization eventually hit me - it was a step that needed to be taken. With a heavy heart, I reached out to my family and explained that I was fully immersed in my college degree. I let them know that while I would check in occasionally, I could not be available immediately. The first few weeks were undoubtedly tricky. When family members called seeking advice or help, it tore at my heart to gently decline, explaining that I needed to focus on my studies. It wasn't easy, but I firmly expressed, "I'm sorry, I cannot assist right now. I need to get back to my project. Can we discuss this another time?"

Gradually, the dynamics started to shift. I distanced myself from situations that no longer served me, and that is when I started prioritizing my growth. I took charge of my boundaries at work, clearly defining my work hours and creating a separation between my professional and personal life (post-Covid, of course). This separation allowed me to be fully present in each domain, leading to a more balanced and fulfilling existence.

Food Boundaries

Many of us find it hard to set limits when it comes to food - we love to indulge! Do not get me wrong; the occasional treat is okay. The trouble arises when we need clear boundaries with our food choices. However, I am here to guide you and help you flex those boundary-setting muscles when it comes to what you eat.

Let us take a moment to understand the food industry's game plan. The objective is to make products not just tasty but almost irresistible. The food industry has figured out the perfect formula to light up our brain's pleasure centers, making us want to devour the entire container and then some. And guess what? You find yourself going back for more mouthwatering treats time and time again.

I get it; sometimes, you might want to cut back on certain foods, but it feels like an uphill battle. That is because chemicals strategically added to the food make it incredibly hard to resist. They create a pull that's difficult to break away from. When you try to step back, you might even experience withdrawal symptoms, which only add to the challenge. It is a powerful reminder that it is not just about willpower - there are tangible factors at play that can influence your eating habits.

With consistent effort, you will find that these practices become second nature, supporting your journey towards a balanced and nourishing diet to establish a healthier relationship with food, one on mindfulness and self-awareness. Setting and maintaining healthy food boundaries is essential to developing a better relationship with food and maintaining a balanced and mindful approach to nutrition. Here are some tips for establishing and sticking to food boundaries:

Define Your Boundaries: Clearly outline what your food boundaries are. This could include specific dietary choices, portion control, or guidelines for certain situations (e.g., social gatherings and holidays).

Eating a nutritious snack before an event primes your body for better nutritional choices. It stabilizes blood sugar levels, providing sustained energy and preventing impulsive decisions. This practice jumpstarts metabolism and readies your digestive system, ensuring optimal nutrient absorption from subsequent meals; this leads to a positive, mindful approach to eating, enhancing the dining experience. Pre-event snacking empowers you to align food choices with your health goals, promoting vitality and fulfillment.

Understand Your Triggers: It is essential to clearly understand the triggers that may cause you to deviate from the boundaries you have set for yourself. Identify situations, emotions, or environments that can trigger you and become aware of them. To manage these challenges, gaining insight into your thought processes and behaviors is crucial. Being mindful of your triggers can help you stay in control and make better decisions in adversity.

Communicate Your Boundaries: It is important to communicate your boundaries regarding food preferences, especially if you are in a social setting or living with others. You can set expectations and avoid unnecessary temptations by expressing your needs clearly and assertively. This can help create a more harmonious and respectful environment for everyone involved.

Plan Ahead: One of the keys to maintaining a healthy diet is to prepare meals and snacks in advance. By planning and having healthy options readily available, you can significantly reduce the likelihood of making impulsive, less healthy choices; this saves time and money and ensures that you are fueling your body with nutritious meals and snacks throughout the day.

Practice Mindful Eating: One way to maintain a healthy relationship with food is to practice mindful eating. This involves paying close attention to your body's hunger and fullness cues. Focusing on being present in the moment makes you more aware of your body's signals, allowing you to recognize if you are still hungry and have enough to eat. This can help prevent overeating and promote a more balanced and enjoyable eating experience.

Learning to Say No Gracefully is an essential aspect of self-care. It is perfectly okay to politely decline when offered food that does not align with your dietary restrictions or personal preferences. You do not have to justify your choices to others or feel guilty about them. Remember that saying no is a form of self-respect and helps you maintain healthy boundaries. Being assertive yet respectful can effectively communicate your needs and avoid compromising your health with dietary options that no longer align with you.

Have Alternatives Ready: It is always a good idea to be prepared in case your preferred food choices are unavailable. This is especially important when you have certain boundaries that you want to maintain. Therefore, it's recommended to have some alternative options that are still in line with your dietary restrictions or preferences. This way, you can avoid making impulsive decisions that may not be the best for your health.

Avoid Extreme Restrictions: Extreme restrictions can make you feel deprived and ultimately hinder your progress. Strive to make healthy choices and allow yourself to enjoy the foods you love in moderation. This way, you can maintain a healthy relationship with food and sustainably achieve your goals.

Seek Support and Accountability: Share your food boundaries with a trusted friend or family member who can provide encouragement and hold you accountable. My accountability patterner is my daughter; she loves to call me out when I do not make healthier choices; her favorite phrase is, "Mom, I do not want to hear you complaining when you get pimples after you eat THAT!"

Practice Self-compassion: Be kind to yourself if you slip up. It is expected to face challenges in maintaining food boundaries. Use it as an opportunity to learn and grow. I used to punish myself at the gym after making less healthy food choices. I would extend my workout routines because of an indulgence. However, when I started being kinder to myself, I flourished in my health journey. I started reminding myself that it is a process, and I will make healthier choices at the next meal because I cherish how I feel when I nourish my body with wholesome foods. I have become attuned to my body's reactions to both healthy and less healthy meals, and my body favors the healthier options.

Reflect and Adjust: Take some time to periodically reflect on your food boundaries. Life is constantly changing, and so are your needs and circumstances. Therefore, it is necessary to establish food boundaries that align with your individual health objectives and lifestyle. By being mindful of your food boundaries and making necessary changes, you can achieve your health goals. It is important to have appropriate portion sizes according to your body and nutritional needs so that you don't overeat or undereat. Your stomach is the size of your fist, so it is important to avoid consuming too many unhealthy foods and snacks or any large amount of food. Gradually reducing your sugar and sugary soft drink intake is also a good idea. Pay attention to your body's hunger and satiation levels and respect them. If you are eating out and reach your satiety level but still have leftovers, don't hesitate to ask the server for a to-go container or ask them to take away the food. If the food is still in front of you, you may be tempted to continue eating beyond your satiety level.

Drinking Boundaries

Establishing boundaries around what you drink is a significant step towards a healthier lifestyle. This applies to soft and sports drinks and caffeinated and alcoholic beverages. While they can be a refreshing treat, be mindful of your consumption. Many of these beverages are packed with sugars and additives that can challenge your body's natural balance. For instance, a typical 12-ounce soft drink contains a staggering 39 grams of sugar, equivalent to about 9.5 teaspoons. Some even contain around 56 grams, roughly 14 teaspoons of sugar! The excess sugars can strain your organs as they work hard to regulate your internal environment. Not to mention the high carbohydrate count in many products, the body converts these carbs into glucose, which can then overload the liver and pancreas.

Do not let deceitful companies persuade you with labels like "diet" or "sugar-free." Surprisingly, some of these options might be different from the healthier choice. They can potentially contain artificial additives and chemicals that challenge your body's natural detoxification processes. Always remember, it is not just about what a product claims to be but about understanding its composition and how it interacts with your body's physiology.

Many diet products use artificial sweeteners like aspartame, saccharin, or sucralose to replace sugar. While these additives are low in calories, they can lead to cravings for sweeter and higher-calorie foods. Over time, this can disrupt your body's natural ability to regulate its calorie intake, potentially leading to overeating. Regularly consuming artificial sweeteners can alter your taste preferences. You might develop a heightened sensitivity to sweetness, making naturally sweet foods like fruits less appealing. This can limit the variety of nutrients you get from your diet. While research on artificial sweeteners is ongoing, some studies have suggested potential links to various health concerns, including metabolic syndrome, altered gut health, and even weight gain in specific individuals.

The body processes many artificial sweeteners as foreign substances. While regulatory agencies generally recognize them as safe, there is ongoing debate about their long-term effects, especially when consumed in large quantities. In addition, research suggests that artificial sweeteners may affect our metabolism. They can alter the composition of our gut microbiota, which plays a crucial role in digestion and metabolism. This disruption can change how our bodies process and store sugars and fats.

Some "sugar-free" products may not contain traditional sugars, but they often have alternative sweeteners or additives that serve a similar purpose. These can have metabolic effects and be problematic for people with sensitive digestive systems. Moreover, certain sugar substitutes can cause digestive discomfort in some individuals. They may lead to symptoms like bloating, gas, or even diarrhea.

Considering all these factors, it is important to approach "diet" and "sugar-free" products with a discerning eye. Reading ingredient labels, understanding the potential impacts on your body, and listening to your bodily reactions can be critical steps in making informed dietary choices.

7 Strategies to Optimize Your Health & Prevent Chronic Illnesses.

Opting for whole, minimally processed foods whenever possible is often the best way to support your body and optimize your health.

Regarding caffeine, I am not suggesting you give up your morning coffee if you are an avid coffee drinker (I would not dare!). As coffee drinkers, we rely on that burst of sugar and caffeine to get through the day. However, limiting your intake of caffeinated beverages to 8 ounces per day is advisable. If you need a second boost, opting for a caffeine-free alternative is best. It is essential to note that even products labeled as "caffeine-free" may contain trace amounts of caffeine. Similarly, the "sugar-free" label can be misleading, as such products may contain sugar under a different name. With over 100 names for sugar, it is crucial not to be deceived by labels.

The truth is that the healthier your lifestyle, the more natural energy your body will generate. Adopting nutritious eating and sleeping habits naturally diminishes your reliance on caffeine. Your body will thank you for it as it thrives on nourishing, wholesome practices.

Increased caffeine intake can have a range of effects on the body. Some individuals may experience difficulty sleeping, leading to insomnia or disrupted sleep patterns. This can result in feelings of restlessness and shakiness, as well as heightened levels of anxiety. Physiologically, higher caffeine consumption can lead to an elevated heart rate, potentially manifesting as arrhythmia or a fast heart rate. It may also cause muscle tremors and increased blood pressure. Digestive issues are also a common occurrence, with symptoms such as diarrhea and upset stomach being reported. In some cases, excessive caffeine intake can lead to dehydration, which may exacerbate other symptoms. Headaches, nausea, and dizziness are additional potential side effects. It is important to be mindful of these symptoms and consider moderating caffeine intake to mitigate their occurrence. If any of these effects become severe or persistent, seeking medical advice is recommended.

Increased caffeine intake can lead to difficulty sleeping, anxiety, arrhythmias (abnormal heart rate, typically increased heart rate), muscle tremors, high blood pressure, dizziness, diarrhea, upset stomach, dehydration, restlessness/shakiness, headaches, nausea, and, at times, increased caffeine can cause slippiness (not too common). Did you know withdrawal symptoms from caffeine and sugar are similar? These symptoms include mental fog, irritability, headaches, nausea, and drowsiness.

Setting boundaries with what you consume isn't about deprivation; it is about empowering yourself to make choices. Your body, mind, and spirit will thank you for it in the long run.

Gradually reducing caffeine intake is key to a successful transition. I vividly recall my initial attempt to quit coffee during my sophomore year in college. My daughter was just 2 or 3 years old then, and we were on vacation to the Dominican Republic to visit my mother, who lived there then. Little did I know this decision would lead to a transformative experience. For an entire week, I found myself confined to my bed. I'd muster the energy to shower, but meals were brought to me by my concerned mother, who was understandably worried about my well-being. I persisted, determined to break free from coffee dependency. However, the process proved more arduous than anticipated, stretching into an entire week. My abrupt cessation of caffeine left me feeling drained and fatigued.

Reflecting on that experience, I now recognize the importance of a gradual transition. It is a lesson I wish I had learned sooner. Nevertheless, the "cold turkey" quitting holds for some individuals. The journey towards reduced caffeine intake is just one facet of a broader commitment to holistic well-being. Progress may be gradual, but every step counts toward your dedication to live the healthiest life possible.

Alcoholic Beverages

Back in 2011, I used to work with TBI patients (Traumatic Brain Injuries). One of my duties was to accompany patients to AA (Alcoholics Anonymous) meetings. It was profound to witness the impact that alcoholism has on people's lives. I heard multiple stories about how alcohol addiction had wreaked havoc in people's lives. Later, I came to understand how these individuals were using alcohol as a numbing agent to avoid dealing with life's traumas. After all, alcohol is legal, cheap, and quickly provides a temporary escape from the problem. However, the real issue arises with its decreased effectiveness once the alcohol has metabolized, leading to increased consumption at the expense of the liver.

Excessive alcohol consumption can have far-reaching detrimental effects on both physical and mental health. Prolonged and heavy drinking can lead to severe liver conditions, including fatty liver, alcoholic hepatitis, and cirrhosis. It also poses a risk to cardiovascular health, potentially causing high blood pressure, irregular heartbeats, and increasing the likelihood of heart disease.

Chronic alcohol use can result in significant brain damage, leading to cognitive impairments, memory problems, and even neurological disorders. Additionally, it can exacerbate existing mental health conditions and contribute to the development of disorders like depression, anxiety, and substance use disorders. Moreover, high alcohol consumption interferes with nutrient absorption, leading to potential deficiencies, weakening the immune system, and can strain relationships, causing social and interpersonal issues. Heavy alcohol consumption is associated with an increased risk of various types of cancer. Given these potential risks, it is crucial to be mindful of alcohol consumption habits and seek support if needed from healthcare professionals or support groups, emphasizing moderation and responsible consumption.

A Real-Life Story: The Cycle of Alcoholism

In my days as an admission nurse, I admitted hundreds of patients in different healthcare settings. Any healthcare admission is a lengthy process, one that I used to enjoy, except for all the tedious paperwork involved.

One of the cases that will forever stay with me is that of the first Native American patient I cared for. This case, while specific to this individual, is unfortunately not isolated from this cultural background. It reflects a broader pattern seen in cases worldwide, transcending culture and ethnicity.

Common denominators often include a cycle of poverty, alcohol abuse, and a lack of education from one generation to the next. The patient's primary diagnosis was Liver Disease related to alcoholic Cirrhosis stage 3. He had over ten comorbidities and was sent from the local hospital without being stable enough for discharge. The hospitals were overflowing, lacking beds to care for less critical patients. Initially, this patient was supposed to be admitted to home health the day he was discharged from the hospital. However, the company could not reach him, and he did not return the calls promptly. Thus, he was added to my schedule for the following day.

I attempted to reach the patient multiple times before heading to his location, which was not in the safest neighborhood and not a place I wanted to go in the first place. However, this severely ill patient needed medical care as soon as possible. I decided to start the nearly 2-hour drive to see him. I called and left a voicemail announcing my ETA (estimated time of arrival). I had to be strategic about my timing to fulfill my duty as a nurse and not jeopardize my safety.

When I arrived at his house, I thought I had seen it all, but this situation proved me wrong. After knocking on his door repeatedly with no answer, I decided to walk around the house and knock on the windows. Eventually, I heard a faint voice say, "Give me a few minutes." After a short wait, I was greeted at the door by a drunken, shirtless man in his early 60s. He was wearing disposable underwear that was soaked with urine, emitting a strong smell that indicated it had been there since the previous night. As I began assessing this patient, the pungent body odor was overwhelming.

I gently asked him when the last time was, he had a shower. He replied that he did not remember, explaining he had been hospitalized for over a month and did not receive a shower during his hospital stay due to a lack of trust in the hospital staff.

He asked me, "Do I stink that bad?" I replied, "Honestly, your body odor is quite strong, and a freshen-up may help you feel better." He agreed, so I set up a basin with warm water and soap. While he was sponge bathing, I took the opportunity to start my assessment and documentation.

His knees suddenly buckled as he stood up to change into a pair of fresh, clean underwear. I rushed to help him sit back down to prevent him from hitting the floor. He confessed that he had fallen three times that same day and had managed to get up every time after a few hours. This prompted me to ask about his alcohol intake, as the hospital records stated he had been sober for two decades. This opened Pandora's box. Nearly in tears, he explained his pride in his sobriety, considering it a significant achievement. He went on to recount his difficult childhood and how his father had alcohol dependency.

He could not recall a time when his father was sober. He admitted to starting alcohol at around 12 years old and shared about growing up on a nearby Indian reservation. In his forties, he decided to go to rehabilitation, determined not to spend the rest of his life as an alcoholic. He emphasized his pride in this accomplishment, detailing how he worked hard and, with government assistance, acquired a house. He was thrilled to help others leave the reservation and stay with him in the city to find jobs and lead better lives.

He revealed that his alcohol relapse began when the Covid-19 pandemic hit. He felt it was impossible to get sober again and expressed a desire to be no longer alive. However, he lacked the courage to take matters into his own hands and asked if I could assist him. I explained that I became a nurse to save lives, not the other way around, and clarified that I would need to document this conversation in my notes. He nodded in understanding. I told him that if he continued drinking in this manner, it would not be long before his wish came true. I warned him that the disease process would not be easy and that he would not be able to continue helping others in the same way. He listened with wide eyes, asking me questions about possible outcomes.

I smiled and assured him that even though he was drunk and likely would not remember our conversation, I would do my job and educate him. He drunkenly laughed and showed interest in what I had to say. I decided to provide him with a thorough education, knowing that I could not rest that night if I did not go above and beyond to teach this patient, as is my usual approach.

In the end, I focused my teachings on the importance of returning to rehab to get sober again. I scheduled him for the next day to confirm my suspicions that he likely would not remember our previous conversation and might not even recognize me. As usual, I called with my ETA and drove to the patient's house. However, this time, I received no response. A neighbor informed me that the patient had left early that morning to check himself into an in-patient rehabilitation center to get sober. I was beyond surprised. Though my ego took a hit, I realized that I had done what was right. When I got back into my car, all I could say was "HOLY SH*T."

Ready for a confession? Until 2022, I did not know about Indian reservations. Due to my profound lack of American history knowledge (in my defense, that is not something we learn in schools in the Dominican Republic, where I pursued my studies up to college), I believed that the Native American population had vanished from the Earth after Colonization. However, to my surprise, I learned this was not true. I was astounded when I spent time with them. I learned so much from their stories, culture, pain, happiness, and joy. But those are tales from another book.

Tips for Safe Drinking (If Needed)

It's a wise practice to drink water along with alcoholic beverages to stay hydrated. Alcohol can cause dehydration, so replenishing with water can help maintain proper bodily functions and reduce the potential adverse effects of alcohol. Staying adequately hydrated can help you enjoy your social activities while prioritizing your health. So, it's recommended to drink a minimum of 4-8 ounces of water for every drink you consume. Additionally, you can enjoy alcoholic beverages responsibly by ensuring that you eat before, during, and after drinking to ensure proper alcohol absorption and provide a protective buffer. It's also important to have a designated driver to ensure everyone gets home safely. If you don't have a designated driver, you can choose a taxi ride app such as Uber, Lyft, or any other safe ride. Remember, prioritizing your health and safety is always the golden rule when it comes to drinking alcohol.

The following is a story about my first experience in Dubai. I was fascinated by the new world I found myself in where certain actions that might be considered normal in other countries could land you in jail there. One night, I took a taxi ride (I can't recall if it was a regular taxi or an Uber) with a friendly driver. We chatted and laughed about a guy who had tried to get my attention earlier. After a night of heavy partying, I was on my way back to my hotel as the sun began to rise. Feeling extremely tired, my eyes closed for a few seconds when I heard the driver express concern, "Habibti, don't sleep in the car. Sleeping in any public car or transportation can get you arrested here, habibti." This made me curious about what else was illegal in Dubai, and I ended up learning a lot! Habibti is an Arabic common expression of love used for females, for males is called "Habibi."

Please keep in mind the following advice to ensure responsible drinking. It's easy to fall into the trap of salty snacks while drinking but be cautious. Consuming salty treats may lead to drinking more alcohol than intended.

Choose wisely by opting for alcoholic beverages with lower alcohol content. This will enable you to enjoy the occasion without overwhelming your system. Take time to savor your drink and sip slowly. Not only does this enhance your experience, but it also ensures that you are in control of the situation.

Keep track of your drinks to prevent unintentional indulgence. If possible, avoid drinking games, as they can be fun but may not allow you to enjoy your drinks at your own pace.

Remember, responsible drinking means enjoying the moment without compromising your safety and the safety of others.

Storytime: The Wise Grapevine

A wise old grapevine named Vino stood once upon a vineyard nestled between a thermal belt. Vino was known for his sagacity and the wisdom he shared with the grapevines around him.

One sunny day, a young grapevine named Grapie came to Vino, seeking guidance. "Vino," she began, "I have heard whispers about the golden nectar humans create from our grapes. I wonder, should I strive to bear the sweetest fruit?"

Vino, with a twinkle in his leaves, nodded thoughtfully. "Dear Grapie, it is true that our fruits are turned into a delightful elixir enjoyed by many. However, it's essential to remember that balance is the key to a fruitful life."

Grapie looked puzzled. "Balance, Vino? What do you mean?"

Vino began to explain. "Imagine if we focused solely on producing the sweetest grapes. We might neglect our roots, our leaves, and the very soil that sustains us. In doing so, we would become imbalanced, and our health would suffer."

Grapie's eyes widened in understanding. "So, it is not just about being sweet, but about being strong and healthy too?"

"Exactly, dear Grapie," Vino affirmed. "Remember, strength lies in knowing your limits and setting boundaries. You must balance the sweetness with nourishment, ensuring your roots grow deep and your leaves reach high."

Grapie was amazed by Vino's words and began to grow with purpose. She tended to her roots, soaking up nutrients from the soil. She spread her leaves wide, basking in the sunlight, and worked harmoniously with the other grapevines.

As the seasons passed, Grapie's grapes grew plump and full, exuding a perfect blend of sweetness and balance. When harvest time arrived, the humans were amazed at the bounty she offered.

Word of Grapie's wisdom and balanced approach spread throughout the vineyard. Many grapevines followed her example, finding that a well-lived life was not just about being the sweetest but the strongest and most vibrant they could be.

Thus, the vineyard flourished, thanks to Vino's timeless wisdom and Gracie's understanding of balance. Their story became a legend, reminding all grapevines that true fulfillment comes from nurturing every aspect of oneself and that in doing so, they can yield the sweetest, most robust fruits of all. The end!

Social Media Boundaries

Social media and the internet have undeniably revolutionized how we access information, connect with friends, and loved ones, and even indulge in some retail therapy. It is easy to get lost in the endless scroll, especially with algorithms designed to cater to our interests. This can be both addictive and time-consuming, often leaving us wondering where the hours went.

However, it's essential to pause and reflect:

How much of your day is spent in this digital world?

_____

Are you accomplishing all you set out to do?

_____

To help you regain control, I give you five practical tips for setting boundaries with the digital world. First and foremost, be patient with yourself. Breaking free from these well-designed algorithms to keep you hooked to the screen might not happen overnight. Journaling your progress can be incredibly insightful. Each small step forward is a significant achievement. Embrace this journey of social media and internet detox, and you will be amazed at the positive impact it can have on your productivity and possibly cash savings from targeted ads that lead you to purchase products you may not even need.

Disable Social Media Notifications: Initially, this might induce a sense of anxiety. However, as you resist the urge to check your phone incessantly, you'll gradually desensitize to the notifications. This leads to increased ease and reduced anxiety in the long term. Take control of your social media, don't let it control you. Keeping notifications off can significantly decrease stress levels.

Implement 21-Day Intervals: Allocate one hour for social media every three hours. This might be challenging at first, but the rewards are worth it. You oversee your phone, not the other way around. Utilize features like Screen Time on iPhones to set daily limits on apps. Android users can use Digital Wellbeing in settings. Keep trying until you master this step.

Progress to 30-Minute Intervals: Extend the time between social media sessions to four hours. It may seem daunting, but believe me, it is achievable. With each milestone, you will gain a sense of empowerment. Utilize the extra time for non-screen activities like reading, going for walks, or engaging in hobbies.

Limit to One Hour Daily: This step is pivotal. Convince yourself that it's doable and you have already won half the battle. Should you stumble along the way, do not be disheartened. Consistency is key.

Mindful Engagement: When you do engage with social media, make it purposeful. Set specific intentions for your time online, such as connecting with friends or seeking out informative content to help you align with your goals. Avoid mindless scrolling but choose a day and time to be flexible and scroll the hours away if needed.

By gradually implementing these steps, you're reclaiming your time and attention from the digital world. Progress may not always be linear, but each effort counts. Stay committed to the journey!

7 Strategies to Optimize Your Health & Prevent Chronic Illnesses.

Relationship Boundaries

Relationships span a vast range, including those with family, friends, and romantic partners. It is crucial to establish boundaries, regardless of the nature of the relationship. Even if you have yet to do so, there is always time to start. While communicating openly is essential, more is needed to rely on words alone. To make a significant impact, you need a clear action plan. Most importantly, you must be the first to respect and enforce your boundaries.

Initially, some individuals may be resistant, but maintaining consistency is key. Eventually, they will recognize the sincerity behind your boundaries and will adapt. If they do not respect your boundaries, ask yourself: Does this relationship/friendship/acquittance align with the person I am becoming? Do I want this person in my life who does not respect my boundaries? It's not just about speaking your truth but embodying it and being truthful and committed to yourself.

Family Boundaries

Often, family relationships can become tangled in a web of unspoken expectations and blurred boundaries. This can lead to detachment, an emotional chill, and even a loss of connection during pivotal family occasions. In my personal journey and professional career, navigating family dynamics has been a prominent challenge. There were moments when engaging with certain family members would dredge up the less admirable aspects of my personality. Balancing the demands of work and school left me emotionally drained after these interactions. Then, I recognized the imperative need to set unequivocal boundaries to define what I could and could not undertake. I candidly communicated my situation, emphasizing my limited availability except in emergencies. This prompted a shift towards self-sufficiency among my family members, close friends, and acquaintances.

Within households where respect is lacking, the strain on relationships intensifies. In my own family, my father took the initiative to hold family meetings, providing a platform to address ongoing issues. These sessions, characterized by spirited debates and passionate exchanges, were pivotal in shaping our familial dynamics.

Self-preservation is not synonymous with abandonment. There are instances where distancing yourself from energy-draining family relationships becomes necessary. Prioritize your healing process, as it lays the foundation for healthier interactions in the future. This does not entail disappearing entirely but rather creating space to regain balance.

In my journey, my relationship with my mother hit rock bottom during my formative years. As the family's perceived "black sheep," I weathered the storm of judgment and misunderstanding. I have embraced this role through my healing journey, recognizing that every experience has led me to my present self. This process paved the way for a more authentic connection with my mother and family. With fresh clarity, I have discarded filters, choosing instead to express myself honestly and respectfully. If a situation weighs on me, I address it directly, whether face-to-face or over the phone, eschewing gossip, and secrecy. This shift towards open communication has been transformative in redefining the dynamics of my family relationships.

Friends and Boundaries

I vividly recall multiple instances where I failed to establish boundaries with friends. This led me into situations that left me feeling deeply uncomfortable, like when I accompanied a friend on a mission to spy on her boyfriend at his workplace. The real issue was not the act itself but rather the knowledge that she was determined to remain in the relationship regardless of his actions. It was disheartening to witness the abuse she endured at his hands. This friendship became emotionally draining, as she chose to stay tied up to her abuser despite the absence of children or shared assets.

Eventually, I decided to create distance, offering one last piece of advice before parting ways. A few years later, we reconnected through social media, and to my delight, I discovered she was now happily married to someone else, with a baby on the way.

Recognizing when a friendship becomes a one-way street, with one party consistently taking advantage, is crucial. In such cases, it is acceptable but essential to step back for your well-being. Toxic friendships can erode your mental health, and it is entirely justified to sever ties for good. Through personal experience, I have learned to relish my own company, even venturing alone, and traveling the world mainly on solo trips. While the initial outings felt somewhat peculiar, I have grown accustomed to and now relish my company.

Consider what you stand to gain by distancing yourself from a detrimental friendship. As you invest in self-improvement and continue your educational journey, you may find it increasingly challenging to maintain connections with individuals who remain stagnant, mentally, spiritually, and financially. In such cases, I encourage you to seek out like-minded individuals. Reflect on where you can find such kindred spirits and take steps to connect safely. with them. Aligning yourself with individuals who share your values and aspirations can be profoundly rewarding in your personal growth journey.

Storytime: The Wise Willow

Once upon a time, a tall and wise willow tree named Osier stood in a lush, vibrant forest. She was known around the globe for her wisdom and ability to offer sound advice to the creatures of the forest.

One sunny morning, as the golden rays filtered through the leaves, a young, spirited rabbit named Huckleberry approached Osier. With eager eyes, Huckleberry sought her guidance on friendship and boundaries.

"Dear Osier," Huckleberry began, "I have friends who often ask too much of me, leaving me drained and unhappy. What should I do?"

Osier gently rocked in the breeze, her leaves rustling like a knowing chuckle. "Ah, young Huckleberry, you are not alone in facing this challenge. It is vital to remember that true friendships are built on mutual respect and support."

With a thoughtful expression, Osier shared a story from her ancient branches. She spoke of a forest critter who, out of love, accompanied a friend on a mission that made them uneasy. The friend, however, remained committed to an unhealthy relationship.

"In such moments, dear Huckleberry, it is crucial to recognize when a friendship becomes a one-way path," advised Osier. "A friend should be someone who uplifts and supports you, just as you do for them."

Eager to learn more, Huckleberry asked, "But how can I protect my well-being without hurting my friend?"

Osier's leaves shimmered like emerald gems as she continued, "Setting boundaries is an act of self-love, my dear. It may be difficult at first, but remember, it is like pruning the branches of a tree to allow for new growth. Your true friends will understand and respect your needs."

Inspired by Osier's wisdom, Huckleberry began a self-love journey by establishing boundaries. Through patience and courage, Huckleberry learned to communicate boundaries, even if it meant stepping back from certain friendships. Over time, new companions entered Huckleberry's life, each one cherishing the values of mutual respect and support.

Thus, the forest flourished, its creatures thriving in a community built on love, respect, and the wisdom of the ancient willow tree, Osier. The tale of the wise willow and the courageous rabbit was shared throughout the forest, a reminder that boundaries, respect, and the shared growth of kindred spirits nurture true friendships. The end!

Work Boundaries

Establishing clear boundaries in the workplace is crucial, especially when it involves personal information and your coworkers' personalities. A guiding principle I follow is only to ask my coworkers questions I would be comfortable answering myself. I generally prefer to keep my private life separate from my professional environment. Of course, I do have a select group of work buddies with whom I occasionally meet outside of work for meals, drinks, or even vacations. However, I'm discerning about whom I let into this inner circle, as I'm cautious about sharing too much about my personal life with coworkers beyond the essentials for casual conversation. While dating a coworker is not inherently wrong, it is not always the ideal scenario. Picture a heated argument at home, only to face your partner at work. The saying "out of sight, out of mind" holds weight here. Having some space allows you to miss your partner and helps to avoid unnecessary gossip among coworkers.

Maintaining professionalism is essential in minimizing workplace drama. Keeping conversations focused on work can save you both time and energy. We spend a significant portion of our time interacting with coworkers; in many ways, they can become like extended family. However, it is important not to let this blur the lines of professionalism.

An open-minded approach, coupled with providing a judgment-free zone, creates a safe and inclusive workplace. Steer clear of workplace rumors and negative discussions about colleagues. You nurture a positive and constructive environment that benefits everyone involved by doing so. Setting boundaries and maintaining professionalism contributes to a healthier work atmosphere and preserves your well-being in the process.

Balancing sharing enough to build trust and maintaining privacy to protect yourself is essential. Remember that every piece of information you disclose can be used in various ways, so it is important to consider what you share and with whom. Being mindful of the details you reveal allows you to control the narrative and present yourself how you want to be perceived. This is especially true in professional settings, where discretion can be an asset.

If a coworker is making you feel uncomfortable, or you feel harassed or bullied, try setting clear boundaries and make the person aware the behavior is not welcomed; if the person continues with the behavior, talk to a supervisor, and if the supervisor does not do anything about it you should continue to escalate the situation by talking to your supervisor's manager.

A thoughtful reminder: Regular breaks, including a dedicated lunch break, are vital for maintaining productivity and optimizing your health. It allows you to recharge and return to tasks with renewed focus and energy. Your future self will indeed appreciate the care you give to your present self.

Boundary Self-Assessment Questionnaire

Introduction: This self-assessment aims to help you evaluate your current boundaries in various aspects of your life. By reflecting on your interactions, relationships, and personal well-being, you can gain valuable insights into areas where you may need to set firmer boundaries or allow more flexibility. Setting and respecting boundaries is a crucial part of maintaining healthy relationships and achieving personal fulfillment.

Instructions: For each statement, please rate how well it applies to you on a scale of 1 to 5, with 1 being "Not at all" and 5 being "Absolutely." Be honest with yourself, as this assessment is for your personal growth.

1. I communicate my needs and preferences clearly to others.
   (1) Not at all (2) Rarely (3) Sometimes (4) Often (5) Absolutely

2. I am comfortable saying "no" when I need to without feeling guilty or obligated.
   (1) Not at all (2) Rarely (3) Sometimes (4) Often (5) Absolutely

3. I prioritize self-care and allocate time for activities that recharge and rejuvenate me.
   (1) Not at all (2) Rarely (3) Sometimes (4) Often (5) Absolutely

7 Strategies to Optimize Your Health & Prevent Chronic Illnesses.

4. I am aware of my emotional limits and communicate them to others when necessary.
    (1) Not at all (2) Rarely (3) Sometimes (4) Often (5) Absolutely

5. I recognize and respect the boundaries set by others in my life.
    (1) Not at all (2) Rarely (3) Sometimes (4) Often (5) Absolutely

6. I am mindful of how certain relationships impact my mental and emotional well-being.
    (1) Not at all (2) Rarely (3) Sometimes (4) Often (5) Absolutely

7. I can assertively express my feelings, thoughts, and concerns constructively.
    (1) Not at all (2) Rarely (3) Sometimes (4) Often (5) Absolutely

8. I can identify situations where I need to set firmer boundaries for my well-being.
    (1) Not at all (2) Rarely (3) Sometimes (4) Often (5) Absolutely

9. I actively practice self-compassion and avoid self-criticism for setting boundaries.
    (1) Not at all (2) Rarely (3) Sometimes (4) Often (5) Absolutely

10. I am open to reevaluating and adjusting my boundaries as my needs and circumstances change.
    (1) Not at all (2) Rarely (3) Sometimes (4) Often (5) Absolutely

Scoring: Add up your scores for all the questions to get your total.
The higher your total score, the more effectively you are currently managing your boundaries.

Interpreting Your Results

- 10 - 20: There may be room for improvement in setting and maintaining boundaries.
- 21 - 30: You have a moderate understanding and practice of boundaries, but there is still room for growth.
- 31 - 40: You demonstrate a good understanding and practice of setting and respecting boundaries.
- 41 - 50: You excel at establishing and maintaining healthy boundaries in various aspects of your life.

This self-assessment is a starting point for self-reflection and personal growth. Use it as a tool to identify areas where you can further develop and strengthen your boundaries.

"You are a masterpiece in motion. Celebrate your unique essence Radiate love and perfection."- Solanyi Ulloa

Chapter 3

Basic Anatomy of the Human Body

The human body is a complex organ system that works together to keep us alive and healthy. To understand how to take care of our bodies, it is important to have a basic understanding of anatomy. Anatomy is the study of the structure of the human body. It includes the study of the bones, muscles, organs, and other tissues. On the other hand, Physiology is studying how the human body works. It includes studying how the different organ systems work together to maintain homeostasis (balance in the body). I will describe these systems with super basic concepts. The human body is made up of eleven organ systems. These body systems are:

Integumentary system: The integumentary system is the most extensive body system, including the skin, hair, and nails. It protects the body from the environment and helps to regulate body temperature.

Musculoskeletal system: The musculoskeletal system includes the bones and muscles of the body. It provides support and structure for the body and allows for movement.

Nervous system: The nervous system is responsible for controlling all the body's functions. It includes the brain, spinal cord, and nerves.

Endocrine system: The endocrine system regulates the body's hormones. *Hormones* are chemicals that travel through the bloodstream and signal different parts of the body to perform certain functions.

Cardiovascular system: The cardiovascular system pumps blood throughout the body to nourish each body system. It includes the heart, blood vessels, and blood. The cardiovascular system pumps blood throughout the body to nourish each body system. It includes the heart, blood vessels, and blood.

Respiratory system: The respiratory system allows us to breathe oxygen in and carbon dioxide out. It includes the lungs, trachea, and bronchi.

Digestive system: The digestive system breaks down food into nutrients the body can use for energy, growth, and repair. It includes the mouth, esophagus, stomach, intestines, and liver.

Urinary system: The urinary system filters waste products from the blood and excretes them from the body in the urine. It includes the kidneys, ureters, bladder, and urethra.

Reproductive system: The reproductive system is responsible for producing offspring. It includes the male and female reproductive organs. The reproductive system is also responsible for producing specific types of hormones.

Lymphatic system: The lymphatic system helps to protect the body from infection and disease. It includes the lymph nodes, lymphatic vessels, and spleen.

Immune system: The immune system is responsible for protecting the body from infection and disease. It includes white blood cells and antibodies.

How the Body Systems Work Together

The body systems work together to maintain homeostasis, or balance, in the body. For example, the digestive system breaks down food into nutrients the body can use for energy. The cardiovascular system then transports these nutrients to the cells throughout the body.

The respiratory system allows us to breathe oxygen in and carbon dioxide out. The oxygen is then transported to the cells in the blood, where it is used to produce energy. The carbon dioxide is then transported back to the lungs and exhaled.

7 Strategies to Optimize Your Health & Prevent Chronic Illnesses.

The endocrine system regulates the body's hormones, which control various functions, such as growth, metabolism, and reproduction.

The nervous system controls all the body's functions, including the other organ systems.

Storytime: The Body's Symphony of Harmony

One serene evening, as the sun painted the sky with hues of gold and lavender, Solange sat beneath her favorite oak tree, engrossed as she dove into a book about the human body. Her interest grew as she read about organs and systems. Solange's heart overflowed with wonder and a deep desire to understand the mysteries of the universe within. As the words danced before her eyes, a gentle slumber embraced her, and she found herself in a wondrous dream.

Solange stood amidst a breathtaking forest in this dream, but something was different. The trees were colossal, their branches intertwined like the keys of a grand piano. She looked down and marveled at her form, realizing she was part of this enchanting symphony.

As she ventured forth, she met a wise old tree, Methuselah, whose branches reached for the heavens, much like the integumentary system that protects the body's delicate and resilient organs. Methuselah's leaves rustled like whispered secrets, and he shared tales of how each system played its part in the balanced harmony of life.

Solange's journey continued, and she encountered the sacred Bhodi Tree, a sapling bursting with vigor and enthusiasm despite being 2,300 years old. The Bhodi Tree's love and compassion showed Solange that the marvelous landscape of the outside world is not much different from the marvelous landscape within the human body. Methuselah yearned to grow as tall and grand as the Pinus Longaeva, the oldest known tree on Earth. Methuselah imparted the wisdom of balance and patience, reminding Solange that true strength was found in steady progress.

Curious and bright, Solange wanted to know beyond the test books how things worked just right with the perfectly orchestrated symphony. She told

Methuselah and the sacred Bhodi Tree, "I want to see inside, to know how the human body works, how it helps us grow."

Then, something magical happened: Methuselah and the sacred Bhodi Tree initiated the symphony of life to show Solange the wonders within the marvelous human anatomy.

Suddenly, she woke up inside herself, a journey through her body, like nothing else, a dream inside of a dream. Within this marvelous dream, Solange started to see how the inner universe within the human body resembles the outer universe of space and time.

She saw skin, hair, and nails, oh so fine, protecting her body like a strong line. Skin cells work hard, always on the mend, and hair and nails are like nature's friend. The integumentary system, a guardian's grace, shielded her essence, a sacred space. Skin kissed by the sun, by breezes laced, a life embraced. In a world inside our skin, there is a special place where our body begins.

Guided by the rhythm of her dream, Solange visited the musculoskeletal system, where bones and muscles wove a graceful ballet of support and movement. Next, the muses of tendons and ligaments danced, a ballet of grace, their symphony entranced. Joints that swayed, a ballet's flight. In the realm of muscles and bones, where veins flow like rivers to call it home,

Solange has a keen, inquisitive heart, a soul of pristine sheen. Obsessed with the cadence and the body's song, she longed to know where this dreamland fair belonged and where skin and marrow wove secrets rare.

Then, Solange went deeper, to the brain's place, where thoughts and feelings find their space. The brain sends messages all around, ensuring our bodies are in good sound. The help of nerves and the spinal cord tells our body what to do. The nervous system, a conductor orchestrating every step, revealed the power of thought, emotion, and motion. Like instruments in an orchestra, each system had its unique melody to contribute. In hidden chambers, neurons spark, and dreams and secrets are wept. The nervous system, conductor's call, orchestrated movement, one and all. In the sanctuary of thought, emotions reside, and consciousness, like a river, glides.

The heart's grand opera began through arteries wide and veins so thin.

A symphony of beats, a pulsing song, life's rich, nutritious blood crimson rivers flowed strong. In chambers of passion, in ventricles deep, a love story, eternally to keep. Hearts are beating in rhythmic time, a love song, the rhythm of life's prime. In sacred chambers, new life did bloom, in nature's waltz, a sacred loom.

The heart, a drummer, steady and true, beats strong rhythms, pushing life through. In warm chambers, where breath did start, the respiratory silk, in alveoli's embrace, the dance of oxygen, life's gentle grace. A ballet of breath, the dance of life's air so fair. Breathing in and out, the lungs do their part, filling us with life, a vital art. Oxygen flows, an orchestrated symphony in our chest, giving us life at its best.

Next, Solange's eyes fluttered wide, a world anew; within her frame, a spectral view of hormones danced in the endocrine show; like messengers, they help us grow and balance the body. They travel through the blood, a unique stream, making sure our body is like a cascade of whispers, a dance of grace, within the glands, a sacred space.

The dance of creation, the rhythm of birth, and the reproductive dance on Earth. A ballet of beginnings, a song of life, in wombs of time, a dance was rife. For life to go on and new tales to be spun, there is a system for ensuring it is done Reproductive organs play a crucial role in making new life and hormonal balance.

Through rivers of twists and turns, a journey long, the digestive's tale, a smooth mouth to belly, a gastronomic dance, the body's feast, a nourishing pulse. A feast takes place in the tummy's world, and the food's journey starts steadily. The stomach and intestines play their part, breaking down food; it is a work of art.

To rivers deep, the kidneys led, in chambers dark, secrets were bred.

A cleansing symphony, a filtration's grace, in the urinary silent space.

A balance, a dance of flow, the body's rhythm, a cleansing glow.

The kidneys, like filters, keep things just right, cleaning our blood day and night. They help remove waste to keep us clear and healthy.

Through vessels fair, a current strong, the lymphatic's dance, a lifelong song.

A ballet of cleansing, a symphony of flow, within the vessels, like a river it flows, fighting off germs, is a life-saving show. A dance of defense, a healing grace, in lymph, the body found its space. It cleans up our body, helps it stay strong, and is a hidden hero.

In chambers, brave warriors stood, the immune's ballet, a dance so good. Soldiers strong, defenders true, in blood and marrow, the battle grew.

A dance of protection, in cells and plasma, the body's fight. The immune system, a brave, valiant crew, protects us from harm; it knows what to do. Like soldiers, they fight in blood and bone, keeping us safe; they are never alone.

A sweet dance of existence, a tale replete. Solange danced through the endocrine, cardiovascular, respiratory, digestive, urinary, reproductive, lymphatic, and immune systems in time. Each system played its role, an essential note in the symphony of existence—the body's ballet, a dance so divine, in every heartbeat, in every line. The body is a wonder and works like a song; every part and bit is never wrong. We will dance through our days in rhythm and rhyme; thanks to our bodies, it is the perfect time.

As the dream gently released its hold, Solange waved goodbye to Methuselah and the sacred Bhodi Tree. Solange awoke beneath her beloved oak tree; she held grace and appreciation in her heart. The forest whispered its secrets, reminding her that just as every system played its part in the body's dance, every creature played a vital role in the forest's symphony.

Solange lived on, teaching generations the timeless lesson of unity, patience, and the beauty that arises when each part plays its unique role in the symphony of existence. With music in motion and poetry's rhyme, let us dance through life in perfect time. So, let us cherish our bodies; they are precious and grand, and they help us stand with every beat. For in every step and refrain, the body's harmonious dance is life's sweetest gain. And so, the forest flourished, resonating with the enchanting melody of life. The end!

We are Different Sameness (WADS)

The human body is one of the most intricately designed living organisms ever. While we share 99.9% of our genetic material, the remaining 0.1% renders us unique individuals with genetic variations such as height, hair color, and eye color.

As human beings, we are all inherently unique, with a vast array of attributes that set us apart from one another. Our differences can include but are not limited to our skin tones, eye and hair colors, body shapes and sizes, habits, cultures, lifestyles, belief systems, religions, socio-economic statuses, and so much more. These characteristics make us unique and contribute to the richness of our society. Acknowledging and celebrating this diversity is essential, as it allows us to understand our world better, learn from one another, and grow individually and collectively. Recognizing and valuing our differences can create a more inclusive and harmonious society where everyone feels seen, heard, and accepted.

With all the differences between us, how can we be the same?

_____

_____

_____

_____

Humanity is a diverse and complex species, yet we share a remarkable similarity in our genetic makeup. There is a 99.1% overlap between individuals, which leads to a host of commonalities that we all share. Our biological makeup equips us with complex systems that work in tandem to maintain and preserve life, such as the cardiovascular, respiratory, digestive, and immune systems. These systems ensure that our fundamental needs are met, such as nourishment, rest, and safety.

Apart from our physiological needs, we are also driven by various emotional needs unique to each individual. These needs range from love and happiness to fear and sadness, significantly influencing our behavior and actions. We possess a keen sense of right and wrong, shaped by our upbringing, culture, and personal beliefs.

Communication is essential to our survival and well-being. We have developed complex languages and systems of communication that allow us to share ideas, thoughts, and emotions with others. Socialization and a sense of belonging are also crucial to our well-being. We are social creatures and thrive when we are part of a community.

Despite our commonalities, each of us is also unique in our capabilities. We possess math, reading, and writing skills that distinguish us from other living creatures. Our ability to think, reason, and problem-solve is unmatched. We have created complex societies, built incredible structures, and explored the far reaches of space. Our potential for growth and development is infinite, and we continue to push the boundaries of what is possible.

Now, let us engage in a quick exercise

Begin by taking five slow, deep breaths through your nose, allowing the air to fill your lungs, and then exhaling through your mouth with a big, relieving exhale. As you do so, let your body relax and your mind clear.

Now, imagine a world where everyone looks exactly the same - the same skin color, the same eye color, the same height, the same body shape. Imagine that everyone has the same food preferences, clothing choices, habits, hobbies, and essentially everything the same. In this world, no sense of individuality exists. There are no unique identities, no peculiarities, and no diversity. It is a world where every street looks the same, every house looks the same, and every person looks the same.

As you envision this world, notice how it makes you feel. Do you feel relieved that you do not have to think about how you look or what you wear? Or do you feel a sense of unease at the thought of losing your individuality?

Take five more slow, deep breaths through your nose and exhale out through your mouth with a big, relieving exhale if your eyes were closed. As you do so, focus on the feeling of the air moving in and out of your body. Take a moment to appreciate the unique person that you are, with your thoughts, feelings, and experiences.

How did this imagined world feel for you?

_____

_____

_____

_____

The world depicted above is a desolate and melancholic place, where the absence of diversity and uniqueness makes it arduous for individuals to form genuine connections and discern one person from another. The uniformity of the surroundings offers no joy, celebration, or appreciation of individuality, and the lack of diversity has led to a monotonous and tedious existence where people are trapped in repetitive cycles, exhibiting the same behavior, and adhering to the same ways of thinking, ultimately resulting in the stagnation of knowledge and progress.

A world that lacks diversity and uniqueness is doomed to fail and is on a path towards extinction. Instead, we must strive to embrace our differences and celebrate the things that make us unique. We should aim to become better versions of ourselves each day rather than aspiring to be someone else, as it undermines the very essence of individuality. Embracing our differences is not a weakness but a strength; only by celebrating diversity and uniqueness can we move toward a brighter and more inclusive future.

Storytime: The Canvas of Uniqueness and Unity

A diverse community of human creatures lived in a mysterious town between gentle slopes. They hailed from different walks of life, each bearing unique traits, customs, and beliefs. Among them was a wise elder named Elder Alden, whose branches extended wide, offering shade and wisdom to all.

One bright morning, a gentle breeze carried whispers of discord through the town. Differences that once enriched their lives now seemed to divide them. Human creatures began to view their varied attributes as barriers rather than blessings.

Witnessing this rift, Elder Alden decided it was time to share a tale of transformation and unity to remind them of their shared roots. Elder Alden gathered the creatures beneath its ancient boughs and began to speak:

"Once upon a time, In the world of Monona, a land much like our own, but a world painted in uniform shades of gray, life flowed with an eerie sameness. The inhabitants, known as Monones, mirrored one another with precision. Every street, every village, every face features - a symphony of perfect uniformity

In this world, there were no quirks, peculiarities, or diversity. Everyone shared the same skin and eyes and stood at the same height. Their days unfolded in scripted precision, from synchronized morning routines to identical evening rituals.

In this sea of similarity, there lived a curious soul named Anaro. Restlessness brewed within him, a yearning for something beyond the expected confines. In the quiet of her heart, Anaro harbored dreams of color, vibrancy, and a world unseen.

One fateful day, while wandering the meticulously groomed streets of Monona, Anaro stumbled upon a forgotten relic - a small, weathered book, its pages whispering secrets of a world once filled with individuality. The book held tales of distant lands where uniqueness was celebrated, and every soul painted their vibrant canvas upon the collage of existence.

As Anaro explored deeper into the book's tales, a spark ignited within him. The stories awakened a longing for something more, something beyond Monona's stifling borders.

Determined, Anaro began to weave threads of deviation into his life quietly. He donned a single, daring splash of color amidst the sea of gray, a bloom of red against the monotony. He explored tastes beyond the prescribed palate, discovering flavors that danced on his tongue like secret melodies.

Word spread like wildfire of Anaro's unconventional ways, and a whisper of intrigue rippled through the hearts of his fellow Monotones. Slowly, tentatively, others began to seek out their whispers of uniqueness, subtle ripples in the sea of sameness.

The monotony began to shift, imperceptibly at first, but then in sweeping waves. It was as if a dormant vitality had been awakened, a thirst for individuality that had long been stifled.

As the once monochrome streets began to bloom with hints of diversity, a beautiful energy pulsed through the veins of Monona. Faces once mirror images now bore traces of distinct character, eyes that held stories, and dreams that dared to break free.

The world began to transform, not into chaos, but into a symphony of harmonious individuality. Each soul painted their vibrant strokes, creating a more wonderful and prosperous environment than they could have imagined.

And so, Monona, once a world of unending sameness, blossomed into a harmonious world where every heartbeat had its unique rhythm. Anaro's courage to seek the extraordinary in the ordinary sparked a revolution of self-expression and celebration of diversity.

The story of Anaro and Monona's transformation echoed through the ages, reminding all who heard it that even in the most uniform of worlds, the seed of individuality lies dormant, waiting for the right touch to awaken it and turn a canvas of sameness into a masterpiece of uniqueness and vitality.

Once Elder Alden finished the story, the human creatures began to focus more on noticing their differences. They saw varying colors, patterns, and textures and felt a sense of unease. They questioned how they could be a part of the same canvas when they were so different. They stated that Anaro's story was great, but now the differences are too extreme to reach a middle ground.

Elder Alden spoke with the community leaders of each tribe; in his final meeting words, he said, "If your species want to survive and thrive among all the species of this planet, you must unite; if rifts and disagreement continue, the extinction of your species will come. I advise you to see Wefan. Tell Wefan I Elder Alden sent you."

The ancient, wise, and compassionate Wefan welcomed them with open arms. His ancient wisdom and compassion optimized his beautiful eyes with gold flecks. Looking into his eyes was like looking into a vast universe and the beauty of its galaxies.

Wefan welcomed them into the simplistic yet cozy cottage. The leaders of the human creatures began to express their concerns about their differences, violence, and uncertainty, and they sought guidance to help them understand how to live harmoniously. So, Wefan is the ancient being known for his wisdom and compassion for centuries. The Wefan listened intently to their concerns and then began to work.

Wefan interlaced the threads with skilled hands, placing them together in a united dance. Strokes of natural colors adorned the canvas. Each thread retained its individuality, yet now they were bound by a shared purpose.

The threads marveled at the emerging intricate patterns as the canvas took shape. They saw how their differences created a more vibrant and beautiful masterpiece than any one thread could be alone.

At that moment, they understood the true power of unity. They realized that their diversity was not a source of division but a source of strength. They celebrated their unique qualities and embraced their shared purpose.

They understood the connection between human creatures and nature's creatures. This interconnectedness brought them harmony and lifted their spirits. Thus, the canvas flourished, symbolizing unity and harmony for future generations.

Wefan fell silent, allowing the story to settle in the hearts of the gathered human creatures. They looked at one another with sharp understanding, recognizing that their differences were not a cause for division but a source of strength.

From that day forward, the town thrived as a united community, celebrating the rich canvas of life that bound them together. They learned that they indeed became one in embracing their loving differences.

Thus, the legacy of unity and acceptance echoed through the hills, reminding all who listened that our shared purpose and appreciation for our unique qualities bring us together in love and harmony. The end!

From birth, we embody the essence of divine beings, reflecting the universal energy that flows through our existence. However, as we journey through life, external forces such as the environment and circumstances can often conspire to obscure this inherent truth. Life's journey is full of twists and turns that can lead us to forget our divine nature. Societal expectations, challenges, and experiences can create illusions that mask our true essence, making it difficult to recognize the divine beauty within ourselves and others. Nevertheless, beneath the many layers of conditioning and societal narratives, the core of our being remains divine, pristine, and untouched by external influences. Recognizing this divine essence within ourselves and others unveils a profound truth that we are all connected to the core of divine design. Embracing our divine nature is not an act of attainment but a process of remembering, peeling away the layers of illusion to reveal the radiant core within. By acknowledging our intrinsic connection to divine design, we reclaim the power to live authentically, guided by the wisdom that flows from our divine source. In essence, life's journey becomes a sacred unveiling, a process of rediscovering the divine masterpiece that we truly are. Through this realization, we transcend the limitations imposed by external influences, embracing the truth that we are, and always have been, divine beings intricately interwoven with cosmic design.

Journaling Time

Please write down your thoughts, insights, AHA moments from chapter 3.

_____

_____

_____

_____

_____

_____

_____

_____

_____

_____

_____

_____

_____

_____

_____

_____

_____

_____

_____

"It is health that is real wealth and not pieces of gold and silver." –
Mahatma Gandhi

Chapter 4

Hydration

Learning objectives

- Importance of Hydration
- Body Systems and Their Needs for Hydration
- Dehydration & How to Identify It.
- Learn to Identify Your Unique Hydration Needs.

Why is Hydration Important?

Every cell, tissue, and organ in our body depends on water to function efficiently. It is like the lifeblood that keeps our bodily systems working in harmony. Water is essential for delivering vital nourishment to every part of our body. It is often referred to as the elixir of life because it plays a significant role in maintaining the delicate balance of our bodily functions. Adequate water intake is not just about quenching your thirst, but also about keeping the complex machinery of your body well-lubricated and in smooth operation. Think of water as the conductor of a grand orchestra, coordinating each instrument.

Moreover, water plays a vital role in purging the body of toxins we encounter daily. These toxins can sneak in through the food we eat, the air we breathe, and even the products we use. Fortunately, with the proper hydration balance—what experts call homeostasis—our bodies can efficiently flush out these unwanted guests and safeguard our inner sanctuary.

Consider your body a magnificent mosaic composed of roughly 75% water, a percentage that varies with age. This watery foundation underscores just how integral hydration is to our very existence. It is the foundation upon which all bodily functions rest, ensuring we can thrive, grow, and live life to its fullest potential. In essence, water is the unacclaimed superhero, quietly supporting the grand opera of our existence. Its absence would disrupt the delicate choreography, leaving our bodies without the life-enabling sustenance they crave. Thus, let us honor this precious elixir, recognizing it not only as a source of life but as the essence that allows us to flourish and thrive.

Average percentages and ranges of water in the body according to sex and age:
Men: 12-18 years 59%, 19-50 years 59%, 51 years and over 56%.
Women: 12-18 years 56%, 19-50 years 50%, 51 years and over 47%.
Infants and children: 74%.

The percentage of water in your body is a dynamic and complex aspect of human physiology. It can vary significantly based on a multitude of factors. One of the key influencers is a person's ethnicity, as different ethnic groups may exhibit varying water composition tendencies. It is a dynamic interplay of genetics, lifestyle, environment, and physiology, highlighting the intricate nature of our biological systems.

Socioeconomic background also plays a role. Access to clean and safe drinking water and the availability of a balanced and nutritious diet can impact one's overall hydration levels. Additionally, body size and shape contribute to this percentage. More prominent individuals, for instance, may have a higher total water content due to their increased surface area.

Muscle mass and fat percentage are crucial determinants. Muscles have a higher water content than fat tissue, meaning individuals with higher muscle mass might have a more significant overall water percentage, requiring more water than the average human. Activity level is another significant factor. Those who engage in regular physical activity may experience higher water content due to the increased demand for hydration during exercise.

Environmental factors also come into play. In hotter climates, individuals may naturally have a higher water content to help regulate body temperature and counteract increased fluid loss through sweating.

The human body is a marvel of biological engineering, often likened to the world's most luxurious and high-performance cars. Just as luxury brands like Lamborghini, Ferrari, Bugatti, and Rolls-Royce boast meticulously designed engines and intricate systems, our bodies testify to luxury, thoughtful design, and seamless functionality. If we were to assign a vehicle designation to the human body, it might be called "GME" (Greatest Machine Ever, and yes, I made that up), pronounced with the flair of Italian and French accent influence.

Nevertheless, let us keep things straightforward

Skin, our body's largest system, is a true testimony to the power of hydration. It contains approximately 64% water, and well-hydrated skin boasts a natural radiance and vitality. Ensuring you are drinking enough quality water suitable to your body type and activity level provides a boon to your skin's health.

Adequate hydration amplifies the body's natural detoxification processes, facilitating the expulsion of toxins more effectively. This surge in blood circulation to the skin cells culminates in smoother, more evenly toned skin. Puffiness is reduced, elasticity is heightened, and wrinkles become less pronounced.

Moreover, maintaining proper hydration is pivotal in balancing the sebaceous glands, which regulate oil production. This, in turn, helps prevent clogged pores—a common precursor to acne. Beyond that, well-hydrated skin is less prone to irritation and itching, ensuring a comfortable and radiant complexion. Prioritizing hydration thus becomes the foundation of nurturing skin health, contributing to its elasticity, supporting a flourishing gut, and minimizing blemishes.

Storytime: The Fountain of Radiance

In a distant land, nestled between emerald forests and azure lakes, a village existed like any other. The inhabitants of this village, known as the Luminae, possessed skin that glowed with an ethereal radiance. Their secret lay in a legendary fountain that graced the heart of their village.

The fountain was said to be a gift from the highest universal supreme being, a source of life-giving waters that bestowed upon the Luminae their luminous complexion. The village prospered under the benevolent glow, and the Luminae thrived in harmony with their surroundings.

One day, a curious Lumina named Ella embarked on a quest to learn more about the fountain's magic. She ventured into the surrounding forests, seeking the wisdom of the ancient trees and creatures. Along her journey, she encountered an old and wise owl named Orion.

With eyes gleaming like the stars, Orion shared the tale of the human body, a marvel of engineering akin to the most beautiful creation of the Milky Way galaxy. He spoke of its intricate systems and their reliance on water for optimal function, likening it to the life-giving essence that flowed from the Luminae's fountain.

Ella's heart swelled with enlightened understanding. She realized that the Luminae's radiant skin was not solely a result of the mystical waters but also co-related to the power of hydration. The fountain was a symbol, a reminder of water's vital role in nurturing their bodies.

Eager to share this revelation with her fellow Luminae, Ella returned to the village, her heart brimming with purpose. She gathered the villagers beneath the ancient trees and spoke of their fable with Orion by her side.

"In the heart of our village lies a fountain, a gift from the highest universal supreme being, a fountain used by our ancestors," Ella began, her voice carrying the weight of enlightened wisdom. "But let us not forget that the true source of our radiance lies within ourselves."

She recounted Orion's tale of the human body, an intricate design, and seamless functionality, much like the most coveted joyous existence. The

91

Luminae listened with rapt attention, their hearts swelling with gratitude for the knowledge bestowed upon them.

From that day forward, the Luminae embraced the wisdom of hydration, recognizing it as their vitality and radiance. They tended their bodies carefully, ensuring they were well-hydrated and nourished.

The village flourished, not just in their skin's glow but in their spirits' vigor. They became an example of health and vitality, the power of understanding and embracing water's simple yet profound role in sustaining their GME (greatest machine ever).

So, the legend of the Fountain of Radiance lived on, not just as a mystical source of water but also as a reminder of the Luminae's innate wisdom and ability to nurture their brilliance from within. The end!

The Marvelous Human Brain

The human brain is an incredible organ made up mostly of water, accounting for about 73% of its entire composition. This fact emphasizes the importance of hydration for optimal cognitive function. When the body does not receive enough water, the brain has to work harder to perform its many tasks, which can result in mental fatigue and a range of other symptoms.

Inadequate hydration significantly impacts mental acuity and overall well-being. The human brain is responsible for many tasks that require a lot of energy, including thinking, processing information, and controlling movement. When the body is dehydrated, the brain must work harder, which can result in decreased cognitive function, poor memory recall, and difficulty concentrating.

Other symptoms of inadequate hydration include headaches, dizziness, confusion, and irritability. These symptoms can be debilitating and interfere with daily activities. Staying hydrated by drinking enough water throughout the day is crucial to maintain optimal cognitive function.

Storytime: The Wise Oliver and the Crystal Stream

In a tranquil forest, there lived a wise man named Oliver. Known for his unparalleled knowledge and keen intellect, he was revered by creatures near and far. One bright morning, as the sunlight pierced through the canopy, Oliver embarked on a quest to uncover the secrets of the mind.

Deep within the forest's heart, he stumbled upon the most beautiful water element made of a crystal-clear stream, its waters glistening like liquid sapphires.

As he gazed into the shimmering depths, a revelation struck him - the brain, that remarkable organ that bestowed him with wisdom, was predominantly composed of water, a staggering 73% of its being.

This knowledge resonated within Oliver, igniting a spark of understanding. He realized that the elixir flowing before him held the key to optimal cognitive function. Without adequate hydration, the brain toiled relentlessly, striving to perform its myriad tasks.

With purpose in his heart, Oliver spread his wings and took flight, seeking to share this revelation with the forest's creatures. He spoke of the profound impact of hydration on mental acuity and well-being, emphasizing the importance of nurturing the body and mind in harmonious unity.

As the forest inhabitants listened to Oliver's wisdom, they were grateful for this understanding. They gathered by the crystal stream, making a pact to prioritize their hydration, knowing it was crucial for their mental prowess.

Thus, the forest thrived in a newfound brilliance, guided by the wisdom of Oliver, the wise owl. His legacy echoed through the trees, a reminder that within the simplest of streams flowed the key to unlocking the mind's full potential. From that day forward, the forest's creatures cherished the crystal stream, for they knew the secret to wisdom, clarity, and boundless possibility lay in its waters. The end!

Circulatory System

The circulatory system of the human body also referred to as the cardiovascular system in medical parlance, is an intricate network primarily consisting of the heart and blood vessels. It is vital in sustaining life by circulating blood throughout the body, nourishing tissues, and eliminating waste products. However, the importance of hydration must be addressed in maintaining a healthy circulatory system. When a person does not consume sufficient water according to their individual needs, it can reduce the volume of blood, thereby affecting the proper functioning of the circulatory system.

Proper hydration is crucial for the smooth functioning of the circulatory system, much like well-maintained engine oil in a vehicle's engine. It facilitates the flow of blood, the life-sustaining fluid, through the veins, arteries, and capillaries, maintaining optimal consistency. When the body is well-hydrated, blood flows smoothly and efficiently, allowing the heart to pump blood with less resistance and reducing its burden. However, dehydration leads to thickening of the blood, making it more viscous and difficult to move. This makes the heart work harder to maintain circulation, leading to higher blood pressure and cardiovascular issues over time if sustained.

Furthermore, proper hydration enhances the flexibility and elasticity of blood vessels. It allows these vessels to expand and contract optimally to accommodate blood flow. However, dehydration can make blood vessels rigid and less responsive, hindering blood flow and putting stress on the heart. Over time, this added stress can increase the risk of developing conditions like high blood pressure and atherosclerosis and even contribute to the formation of blood clots.

Maintaining proper hydration is essential for supporting a healthy circulatory system. It helps keep the network working smoothly, reducing the risk of cardiovascular complications. Prioritizing hydration is a simple yet effective way to keep your heart and blood vessels in top shape, ensuring optimal health and longevity.

Respiratory System

The respiratory system is a complex network that facilitates the exchange of oxygen and carbon dioxide in our bodies. Its efficiency is vital for sustaining life, and optimal hydration ensures smooth operation.

Imagine the cilia (hair-like structure) in your lungs as vigilant sentinels, continuously working to keep your airways clear. When well-hydrated, these microscopic structures can efficiently trap and expel harmful particles, including microbes and foreign substances. This helps maintain clear air passages and acts as a protective mechanism, preventing potentially harmful agents from entering deeper into your respiratory system.

Insufficient hydration, however, can lead to a series of challenges for your respiratory health. When deprived of the necessary water intake, the cilia's effectiveness diminishes, making it harder for them to perform their critical function, resulting in a buildup of mucus and secretions. These accumulated substances can serve as a breeding ground for microbes, increasing the likelihood of infections and inflammatory reactions.

Additionally, the moisture level of the air you breathe is influenced by your hydration status. When adequately hydrated, the respiratory tract can effectively humidify incoming air, ensuring optimal gas exchange in the lungs. However, without enough water, this process becomes compromised, potentially leading to irritation, inflammation, and even damage to the delicate tissues of the respiratory tract. Furthermore, dehydration can exacerbate existing respiratory conditions, such as asthma or chronic obstructive pulmonary disease (COPD). It can amplify symptoms, making it more challenging to manage these conditions effectively.

Maintaining proper hydration is like providing your respiratory system with the lubrication it needs to function optimally. It supports the cilia's sweeping action and facilitates effective moisture exchange. By prioritizing hydration, you are safeguarding your respiratory health and enhancing your system against potential threats.

The average human can survive:

- Up to three weeks without food, provided they are drinking water.
- Up to one week without food.
- About three days without water.

However, without oxygen, the average human will die within minutes, with the average time being four to ten minutes.

When you engage in physical activity, your muscles demand more oxygen, which increases the rate and depth of your breath. The respiratory system is vital in meeting this need, ensuring your muscles receive ample oxygen and expel excess carbon dioxide.

In high-altitude environments with lower oxygen levels, the respiratory system adapts by changing one's breathing rate. This adjustment ensures that one's body receives oxygen despite the reduced atmospheric concentration.

Dehydration can lead to oxygen-related issues in several ways. When you are dehydrated, your blood volume decreases, which means less fluid is available to carry oxygen to your cells. This can lead to reduced oxygen delivery to vital organs and tissues and a decrease in blood pressure. When blood pressure drops, it can reduce perfusion (blood flow) to various organs, which may lead to inadequate oxygen supply.

The respiratory system plays a pivotal role in various aspects of our lives. Smoking, including the use of electronic cigarettes and vapes, introduces harmful substances into the respiratory tract, causing irritation, inflammation, and lung damage, ultimately leading to chronic conditions like chronic bronchitis or emphysema.

In addition, conditions like snoring and sleep apnea are closely tied to the respiratory system, involving disruptions in airflow during sleep that can cause irregular breathing patterns. Dehydration can exacerbate snoring and sleep apnea. When dehydrated, your nose and throat mucus can become stickier and thicker; this can obstruct the airways, making breathing more difficult and increasing the likelihood of snoring. The airways may already be partially blocked in individuals with sleep apnea, and dehydration can worsen this condition. Also, dehydration can lead to dry mouth and throat, further contributing to snoring and sleep apnea episodes.

Deep breathing techniques are invaluable tools in stress management. They involve deliberate, controlled inhalation and exhalation patterns that engage the diaphragm, a crucial muscle responsible for breathing. Individuals can enhance their lung capacity and oxygen intake by consciously activating the diaphragm, promoting a sense of calm and relaxation. This intentional focus on deep, measured breaths helps regulate the body's stress response, reducing feelings of anxiety and promoting a state of mental and physical equilibrium. Moreover, these techniques have far-reaching benefits, impacting stress levels and overall respiratory health, making them a valuable practice for holistic well-being.

Storytime: The Wise Wind and the Curious Creature

Once upon a time, a curious human creature named Azury lived in a land where nature's elements held wisdom. Azury was known for his insatiable thirst for knowledge and his adventurous spirit.

One sunny day, Azury decided to discover the secrets of the elements. He traveled through lush forests, crossed babbling brooks, and climbed towering mountains until he reached the tranquil Valley of Elements.

Azury encountered the Wise Wind in this valley, an ancient and sagacious spirit who knew the world's elements. Azury approached the Wise Wind with humility and asked, "Oh, Wise Wind, can you share with me the mysteries of the elements and how they shape our lives?"

The Wise Wind smiled and agreed to teach Azury through a tale. He began, "There are four great elements: Earth, Water, Fire, and Air. Each plays a vital role, but today, let me tell you the tale of Air, the element that breathes life into every living being."

Azury's eyes widened with intrigue as he listened attentively to the Wise Wind's story.

"In every breath you take," the Wise Wind began, "Air is there to nurture you. It fuels your every step, dance, and leap. It whispers secrets in the rustling leaves, carries seeds to new homes, and paints the sky with vivid hues. Air is the breath of life, connecting all living creatures."

Azury nodded in understanding, realizing the profound significance of the element of Air. He felt appreciation for the Air he breathed and how it sustained him.

As Azury bid farewell to the Wise Wind, he carried this wisdom on his journey. He now understood that every breath he took was a gift, a reminder of the interconnectedness of all living things.

From that day forward, Azury was grateful for the elements, cherishing the Air that gave him life. He shared the tale of the Wise Wind and the element of Air with fellow creatures, inspiring them to appreciate the simple yet extraordinary act of breathing.

And so, in the land where nature's elements held wisdom, the tale of Azury and the Wise Wind became a cherished fable, reminding all who heard it of the precious gift of life's breath. The end!

Digestive System

Your remarkable digestive system comprises ten essential organs. This intricate system relies significantly on adequate hydration to function optimally. Consider, for instance, saliva production, which amounts to approximately 1.5 liters per day. Saliva, a crucial component, initiates the digestive process by breaking down food particles.

Here is a noteworthy point: Many common digestive issues can be mitigated by maintaining proper hydration levels. Picture it as a series of interconnected events when there is insufficient hydration, salivation decreases, impeding the efficient breakdown of ingested foods, exerting additional strain on the stomach, and intensifying its digestive efforts. As a result, the stomach may grapple with processing incompletely broken-down foods; this sets the stage for these inadequately refined food particles to journey into the small intestine, where they face further challenges. Without an adequate water supply, the small intestine encounters difficulties in absorbing nutrients effectively, and this culminates in a cascade of issues, ranging from compromised digestion to suboptimal nutrient absorption, ultimately leading to insufficient nourishment of vital organs.

Moreover, that is not the end of the story. Our expedition concludes in the large intestine, or colon, where hydration again plays a critical role. Inadequate water intake can disrupt regular bowel movements, resulting in constipation, which presents its own set of discomforts and challenges.

Therefore, please consider this: prioritize your hydration. By doing so, you are meeting a fundamental bodily need and ensuring the seamless functioning of your digestive system. A well-hydrated body is akin to a finely tuned machine primed to tackle life's challenges with vitality!

Storytime: The Digestive Dance

Once upon a belly, in a world of munch,
It is a story of digestion. Let us have a hunch.
From breakfast to dinner and all in between,
A dance in your tummy is quite the scene!

From your mouth to your tummy, it is quite a feat.
Organs in action cannot be beaten!
Different cells, doing their part,
Creating a show, a work of art.

The twisty-turny tract, like a roller-coaster ride,
Food's wild adventure, no need to hide!
With twists and turns, it is quite a spree.

Saliva is the starter; in the mouth, it begins,
Mixing and swirling it is where the fun wins!
Chewing and sloshing, creating a ball,
A prelude to feasting, a grand foodie's call!

Down the esophagus, like a slide in a park,
A ride for the bolus, it is quite the lark.
To the stomach, it goes, a chamber so grand,
Where digestion starts to land.

In the stomach's great hall, things heat up,
Bolus turns chyme into a tasty soup.
Acids and enzymes join in the game,
Breaking down food, they are not playing tame!

Gallbladder, liver, and pancreas too,
They are like chefs, cooking up a stew.
They break down the food, making it small.
So, it can be absorbed and used by us all.

Enzymes and hormones, they play a role,
Guiding the process, they are on a roll!
Turning the food into energy so bright,
Keeping us going from morning to night.

To the small intestine, food takes its chance,
Bile joins the party in a digestion dance.
A duet so lovely, they tango and twirl,
Getting things ready for the body's great whirl.

The mesentery is like a big, cozy hug,
Holding things in place, snug as a bug.
Supporting the team, making sure they are fine,
So, they can keep dancing in a perfect line.

Like little fans, Jejunum and ileum absorb nutrients like the biggest of
fans.

They soak up the goodies like a sponge in a sea,
Sending them off where they need to be.
To the large intestine, food makes its way,
Water's drawn out, making things sway.
Into a soft mass called stool, it turns,
Ready to leave, as the body discerns.

Through the rectum, it goes, with a final bow,
It is time to exit, and it takes a bow.
And there you have it, the digestive show,
A tale of the belly, from high to low! The end.

A thriving digestive system typically manifests in daily bowel movements. However, in our modern era, it has unfortunately become commonplace for some individuals to experience bowel movements every 2-3 days, and this is mistakenly perceived as normal. On the other hand, some people may have a bowel movement after every meal, which is considered not only normal but also quite beneficial.

This discrepancy highlights the wide range of what can be considered "normal" regarding bowel movements. It is important to recognize that our bodies are unique, and what is regular for one person may not be the same for another. Therefore, establishing a baseline for what is normal for you is vital to monitor your digestive health.

Moreover, the frequency of bowel movements can be influenced by various factors, including diet, hydration, physical activity, and stress levels. It is essential to maintain a balanced lifestyle to support optimal digestive function. A diet rich in fiber, ample hydration, regular exercise, and effective stress management techniques are all key components in promoting a healthy digestive system. By paying attention to these aspects, you can take proactive steps towards ensuring your digestive health remains in top form.

7 Strategies to Optimize Your Health & Prevent Chronic Illnesses.

Journaling time

When was your last bowel movement?

_____

_____

_____

What was the smell like?

_____

_____

_____

Why do you think it smelled like that?

_____

_____

_____

What can you do to help your digestive system?

_____

_____

_____

The urinary system

The urinary system encompasses the kidneys, renal pelvis, ureters, bladder, and urethra, each contributing to complex functions. The kidneys are remarkable organs predominantly composed of water, constituting about 83% of their composition. Their significance cannot be overstated; they are primary players in the body's detoxification process. After filtering the blood, the kidneys are left with waste products, which they skillfully convert into urine. This urinary mixture is a repository of body toxins, a natural byproduct of the breakdown of foods and medications, supplements, and any substances introduced.

However, the kidneys' responsibilities continue. They act as master regulators for blood pressure, balancing fluids within the body, controlling the production of red blood cells, making vitamin D to help calcium and phosphorus absorption to keep bones healthy, maintaining the body's chemical balance, controlling PH levels, and diligently removing waste and toxins. Additionally, they exert influence over blood pressure.

Let us talk about a common pitfall - not drinking enough water stresses the kidneys, forcing them to work harder to fulfill their vital functions. The consequences of inadequate hydration can be severe, leading to many urinary complications. These may range from recurrent urinary infections to the formation of kidney stones and, in extreme cases, kidney failure.

Proper nutrition and hydration can potentially prevent many of these issues by recognizing the pivotal role of the urinary system and providing it with the support it needs. So, let us raise a glass of good water to the unsung heroes within us - our kidneys! They work tirelessly, day in and day out, to keep us in balance and thriving. Cheers to kidney health!

The endocrine system

The endocrine system is often called the body's internal messenger system. This network of glands, responsible for creating, secreting, and regulating hormones, influences various bodily functions, including sleep patterns, emotional states, cognitive processes, digestion, and intimate desires.

It is crucial to understand that hormonal balance is integral to our health. When imbalances occur, the repercussions can be far-reaching. Heightened stress levels, susceptibility to illness, weight fluctuations, sleep disruptions, and compromised digestion may all manifest as a result.

Proper hydration is crucial here. Without adequate water intake, the endocrine system struggles to maintain hormonal equilibrium. This imbalance places undue strain on the adrenal glands, leading them to overwork in their attempts to compensate. The consequence? Increased fatigue, which can significantly impact daily life.

In essence, nurturing our endocrine system through hydration is akin to tending to the delicate gears of a well-oiled machine. It ensures that our hormones function harmoniously. So, let us raise our glasses of water to the endocrine system, a silent maestro orchestrating the symphony of our health.

Storytime: The Urban Oasis

A remarkable woman named Elana lived in the heart of a crowded city, amidst the ceaseless rhythm of hurried footsteps and honking horns. She was not just an ordinary city dweller; she held within her a profound understanding of the elixir of life - water.

Elana's days were filled with meetings, deadlines, and the constant hum of city life. However, amidst the urban chaos, she carried a secret - a knowledge that could transform lives. She knew that water was the very essence of vitality.

One steamy summer day, as the sun beat down mercilessly on the concrete jungle, Elana found herself in a crowded square. A group of weary commuters surrounded her; their faces were engraved with fatigue and thirst.

With a spark in her eyes and a conviction in her voice, Elana began to tell a tale of the human body systems. She spoke of the digestive, urinary, and endocrine systems, emphasizing their reliance on proper hydration for optimal function. The busy humans listened intently; their hurried steps momentarily stilled.

As the story unfolded, the city seemed to hush, as if nature itself held its breath to hear Elana's words. She painted a vivid picture of how water was not just a mundane necessity but a lifeline that sustained the very essence of their being.

Elana's wisdom resonated with her fellow city dwellers. They realized that amidst the relentless pace of urban life, they had neglected this vital elixir. Water was not just a mundane liquid but the key to unlocking their true potential.

From that day forward, the people of the crowded city became acutely aware of the importance of water. They carried reusable bottles, sought out fountains, and made it a point to stay hydrated amidst their busy lives.

And so, during the crowded city, a transformation took place. Water became a symbol of resilience, vitality, and life itself. The legend of Elana spread to nearby cities as the wisdom of the urban chaos, and in the heart of the city, amidst the hustle and bustle, the urban oasis thrived - a testament to the power of knowledge and the life-giving force of water. The end!

Nervous System

The human body is a remarkable biological machine that relies on a complex system of organs and networks to function correctly. Among these networks is the nervous system, which consists of the brain, spinal cord, and an extensive web of nerves. The nervous system transmits messages and signals throughout the body, enabling us to move, think, and feel. Water plays a vital role in maintaining the health and functionality of the nervous system. It is the anchor that enables seamless communication between the brain, spinal cord, and nerves. Without adequate water intake, the transmission of messages can be impeded, leading to lapses in short-term memory and impaired cognitive function.

Research has shown that dehydration can cause the shrinkage of brain cells, which can lead to a range of issues. In addition to short-term memory lapses, dehydration can impede the ability to relay messages effectively, resulting in slower reaction times and decreased performance in tasks requiring mental acuity. Therefore, staying hydrated throughout the day ensures optimal brain function and focus.

Musculoskeletal System

This system consists of bones, joints, and muscles, each playing an indispensable role in your mobility and support. Bones, those sturdy foundations, are composed of about 31% water. It is water that ensures the nutrients reach their intended destinations. Meanwhile, your muscles, which propel you through life's motions, are astonishingly composed of about 75% water. Hydration is their lifeline, providing the necessary protection and cushioning for tissues, ligaments, and bones. Joints, the masterful architects of flexibility, rely on water to maintain a gel-like cushion known as synovial fluid. This essential fluid serves as a barrier, preventing joints from rubbing painfully against each other. A shortfall in hydration can lead to a decrease in synovial fluid, ultimately resulting in joint discomfort. Hence, quenching your body's thirst for water is not only a favor to your muscular system.

Storytime: The Wise Stream

In a cacophonous city, where the rhythm of life pulsed like a heartbeat, there lived a young woman named Marie. Marie was known for her boundless energy and zest for life, always on the move in a hurry.

One day, Marie felt drained and weary. She rushed through the streets, barely noticing the world around her. She hurriedly passed an old park, curled up in the concrete jungle.

As Marie entered the park, a gentle breeze rustled the leaves of the park trees. Its branches seemed to comfort her. Intrigued, Marie approached, and to her astonishment, she heard a soft, melodic voice emanating from the tree.

"Dear Marie," spoke the tree, "I have watched you rush through life, never pausing to savor the moment. I am the Wise Stream, and I hold the secret to boundless energy and vitality."

Marie's eyes widened in surprise. The Wise Stream continued, "You see, much like you, our bodies are in constant motion, a busy city of their own.

106

Furthermore, like a city, they require a steady flow of nourishment to thrive."

Marie listened intently, captivated by the wisdom of the tree. The Wise Stream shared tales of the body's systems and how they relied on water for optimal function, much like a city needing a steady supply of resources.

As the story unfolded, Marie realized the profound impact of hydration on her vitality. She understood that her body was a marvel, a busy metropolis of cells and organs working in harmony. And at the heart of it all was the Wise Stream, providing the life-giving force that kept everything in motion.

From that day on, Marie learned to slow down, to savor each moment, and to nourish her body with the gift of water. She started radiating energy and life. The city around her seemed to come alive in response, mirroring the vibrancy within her.

Hence, Marie and the Wise Stream echoed through the city, a reminder that amidst the hustle and bustle of life, it is essential to pause, listen, and nourish the body. In doing so, we unlock the boundless energy that propels us through the grand adventure of life. The end!

Storytime: The Guardians Within

In a world teeming with life, a remarkable force is known as the Immune System. These vigilant guardians stand at the forefront, tirelessly defending the body against many infections. It is a complex network of cells, an army ready to act at the first sign of invasion.

Water, the life-giving elixir, is pivotal in the Immune System's ceaseless battle. It is the carrier, the devoted companion of immune cells as they patrol the body, seeking out viruses, bacteria, and foreign germs. Water ensures their swift and efficient travel with each sip, enabling them to respond swiftly to threats.

But water's contribution does not end here. It maintains a delicate balance within the body, allowing immune cells to function at their peak. It facilitates the cleansing process, whisking away the remnants of defeated adversaries and making way for new, resilient cells to take their place.

As the Immune System tirelessly stands guard, it relies on this precious resource to maintain its strength and vitality. Without it, the system is weakened, leaving the body vulnerable to the insidious advances of infections.

The Immune System and its reliance on water is the dance of life within us all. It reminds us that every drop we consume contributes to the battle between health and illness. As a result, in every glass of water, there lay the promise of fortitude, of a strengthened defense against the unseen adversaries that want to breach our walls.

As the Immune System and water's vital role spread, it becomes a reminder of the power we hold within, a reminder that we hold the key to our own resilience and vitality in every drop. The end!

Dehydration

Dehydration, the silent intruder, secretly stresses our bodies, provoking a primal response - the fight or flight mechanism. Like a call to arms, it signals that all is not well and that the body needs rescue.

To truly understand the impact of dehydration, we must venture into mazelike cells, tissues, and organs. Many factors can tip this balance, from fever and excessive heat to exercise and low-carb diets. Even the natural rhythms of life, like exercise, menstruation, and pregnancy, play a role.

In its wisdom, the body expends water through various channels - the skin, the respiratory system, and the kidneys. In dreadful circumstances, it resorts to drastic measures, resorting to vomiting and diarrhea. Medications, too, can influence this delicate dance, with diuretics leading the charge.

Nevertheless, in this, we find a lesson - a lesson in the profound impact of hydration on our well-being. It is a reminder that every sip we take, every drop we consume, contributes to the vitality of our body's performance.

So, let us pay attention to this call to nurture ourselves, to be mindful custodians of our body's most essential needs. In the dance of hydration, we hold the power to maintain the symphony of life in perfect harmony. Drinking the appropriate amount of water for your body type and unique needs is essential to maintaining fluid and electrolyte balance.

Signs and symptoms of mild to moderate dehydration: brain fog, hunger/cravings, irritability, mood swings, increased heart rate, low blood pressure, muscle cramps, headaches/migraine, decreased urine output, dark odor, and unpleasant to urine, constipation, generalized weakness, decreased energy levels causing fatigue and drowsiness, halitosis (bad breath), bloating, dry skin/lips/mouth, new or worsening joint aches and pains, getting sick frequently, heartburn stomach, dry eyes.

Signs and Symptoms of Severe dehydration:

- Increased respiratory rate.
- Increased body temperature may lead to fever.
- Severe dizziness or lightheadedness.
- Unconsciousness or delirium

Sipping water every 1-2 hours is better than chugging a bunch of water simultaneously.

The Balancing Act of Hydration

In the stage of well-being, hydration takes center stage, an undisputed necessity for a thriving body. We have all heard the refrain, "Drink water," a chorus sung in unison throughout this book. Nevertheless, it is crucial to remember that even something as essential as water can be too much of a good thing, mainly if our kidneys are not in prime condition.

Overhydration, though less common than its counterpart, can threaten our health. It is a delicate dance, and our kidneys play the leading role. Generally robust, healthy kidneys can manage the excretion of approximately 1 liter of water per hour. However, when we inundate our system too quickly, the kidneys struggle to keep pace, disrupting the body's delicate balance, a state known as homeostasis. This imbalance can rapidly cause vital electrolyte loss like sodium, a hyponatremia condition.

The signs of overhydration are like subtle warnings, a gentle tap on the shoulder from our bodies. Headaches, nausea, and vomiting may signal that we have crossed the threshold. Meanwhile, the depletion of sodium can lead to a host of symptoms, from coordination issues to overwhelming fatigue and even confusion. In severe cases, it may even lead to convulsions.

However, our bodies are not without their wisdom. Thirst, that primal urge serves as a built-in indicator. Reaching for a drink is your body's way of saying, "I need more."

Now, the question arises: How much water should we be drinking? While some recommend a formula based on weight, it is important to remember that one size does not fit all. The cues our bodies offer are invaluable guides. They whisper when we need to replenish and nudge when we have filled.

In this dance of hydration, let us listen to the music of our bodies, for they are the most astute conductors of this delicate orchestra. In doing so, we find a harmonious and balanced existence.

Personalized Hydration: Listen to Your Body's Tune

Water plays a crucial role in our existence. However, there is no universal score, no one-size-fits-all melody. We each dance to our own rhythm, and our bodies, like astute composers, have unique needs.

The trick is to sip water like a gentle stream, allowing its flow to permeate our day like a steady metronome ticking away the hours—every two hours, a small replenishment based on your body's unique composition. Notice that no set quantity is mentioned here. That is because your body's water requirements are as distinct as your fingerprint, as varied as your individuality.

Knowing your body means understanding its language, whispers, murmurs, and subtle cues. Unfortunately, this truth is often overlooked: we are all different. Our bodies have their own needs and preferences. Water, the elixir of life, emerges as the foremost choice. It nourishes each cell, a vital conduit for flushing out the accumulated toxins of daily life.

Consider the routines that mark your days and the flow of your activities. Are you a sprinter or a marathon runner in this grand race of life? Do you thrive on gentle sips, or do you take hearty gulps? Your body knows best. There is a common refrain: avoid drinking large quantities close to bedtime. Allow your body a peaceful rest, undisturbed by the call of thirst. In this dance of hydration, let us honor our bodies as they orchestrate their own melody, resonating with the rhythm of our cells.

Daily water intake recommendation by age

• Children 1 to 3 years: 1.3 L = 44 ounces
• Children ages 4 to 8: 1.7 L = 57 ounces
• Men ages 9 to 13: 2.4 L = 81 ounces.
• Men ages 14 to 18: 3.3 L = 112 ounces.
• Men 19 years and older: 3.7 L = 125 ounces.
• Women ages 9 to 13: 2.1 L = 78 ounces.
• Women 19 years and older 2.7 L = 91 ounces.

Here's a helpful formula to kickstart your hydration journey: To find your daily hydration goal, simply take your weight (in pounds), divide by 2, and aim to drink that many ounces of water each day. Just remember, this is a starting point because everyone's hydration needs may vary.

The SAC Guide to Optimal Hydration

Paying attention to the details is crucial when striving for optimal health. The acronym SAC, which I created, serves as a guiding star. It illuminates the path to proper hydration and reminds us to listen to our body's whispers every day. Think of it as a checklist for staying healthy.

Smell: The first sentinel is your nose. Freshly voided urine should bear a mild to almost non-existent odor, a gentle testament to your body's balanced hydration. However, should an ammonia-like or strong scent linger, it is a sign. Your body is trying to communicate, suggesting you may be veering into dehydration territory or possibly facing a urinary tract challenge. At this moment, please take note, for it is a call to action. Keep the waters flowing and consult your trusted primary care provider promptly.

Amount: Next, we measure the rhythm of your visits to the "pee pee room." Adequate hydration leads to a steady two-hour cadence, ensuring you visit regularly. Do not be dismayed by these frequent visits; they salute your efficient kidneys at work, safeguarding your hydration.

Color of Your Urine: Your urine is a canvas, revealing the story of your hydration journey. Consult the urine chart below and take note. A pale, straw-like shade signifies you are on the right track, a well-hydrated traveler. A darker urine might signal a need for a little more water in your porcelain throne.

Transparent urine color: overhydrated.

Lemonade urine color: Optimal urine color.

Light beet urine color: Good hydration status.

Amber urine color: You need to drink water.

Burnt orange urine: You are officially dehydrated. Hydrate yourself, preferably with water or electrolytes, without all the sugar and harsh chemicals. Please note that some medications may cause this urine color.

In this dance of hydration, the SAC guide stands as your faithful companion. It reminds you to listen to your body, understand its language, and respond with care. Through these small yet significant checks, you can tune in to what is happening inside your body, allowing you to catch any potential issues before they escalate. These proactive measures play a crucial role in maintaining health. Regular self-assessment empowers you to take charge of your health and address any concerns in their early stages, leading to more effective and timely interventions, ultimately contributing to a longer and healthier life. Your body communicates with you subtly, and attuning to these signals is a powerful tool in safeguarding your hydration.

I created the SAC method mentioned above to educate my patients on their hydration status, so they can be mindful of their urine color, consistency, and smell. You can use the same method, oh and you are welcome!

Sipping to Success: Mastering Hydration Habits

Staying adequately hydrated can be a challenge. Whether you find it hard to drink enough water or struggle with nausea, the following process can help you make hydration a natural part of your routine.

Mind Over Matter: To make hydration a habit, you need to retrain your body's signals. Instead of consciously reminding yourself to drink water, aim to reach a point where your body naturally craves it.

The 21-Day Rule: Creating a new habit takes time and patience. Studies suggest it takes 21 days for the average human to create behavior changes in daily routines. Commit to this journey, and soon, you will find yourself reaching for that water bottle without a second thought.

Set Reminders: During the initial phase, use alarms or notifications to prompt yourself to drink water, which serves as a helpful nudge until your body adapts to the new routine.

Get a Reusable Water Bottle: Having a water bottle within arm's reach makes it convenient to sip throughout the day. Opt for a reusable one; it is eco-friendly and serves as a tangible reminder of your hydration goals. Choose a bottle that helps you tackle the water intake with hours of the day and amount. In-store and online retailers have a great selection; opt for BPA-free and the ones with good reviews.

Infuse Your Water: If plain water is not appealing, add a natural and organic flavor splash. Infuse it with fruits, herbs, or leaves for a refreshing twist. This small change can make a big difference.

Track Your Progress: Keep a hydration journal. Write down how much water you drink each day. This visual record provides a sense of accomplishment and helps you adjust your intake as needed. You can journal in the note section on your iPhone, Google Keep for Android users, or any note-taking app.

Celebrate Milestones: Acknowledge your victories, no matter how small. Celebrate reaching the one-week mark and keep the momentum going. You are on your way to making hydration second nature. Mastering the art of hydration is within your grasp. With dedication and persistence, you will soon find yourself effortlessly meeting your daily water goals. Hydration is not just a habit; it is a journey towards health.

Gradual Hydration: From Juice to Infusion

Fear not if the thought of plain water does not tickle your taste buds! I will share the step-by-step process I followed to help you transition from juices loaded with sugar and chemicals to refreshing infused water. With patience and creativity, you will be hydrated like a pro in no time.

Step Mix It Up with Juice
For the next three weeks, combine half the water with your favorite juice. Pay attention to how your body and taste buds adapt as you sip. If you enjoy the half-water brew sooner, you can move on to the next step.

Step 2: Gradual Dilution
Once you have mastered Step 1, it is time to dilute the juice further. Mix one-third of the juice with water for approximately three weeks. If you still find water a bit of a challenge at the end of this period, extend this step by another week to ease into the transition.

Step 3: Nature's Flavors
Now that you're a pro at dilution, introduce natural flavors. Infuse your water with your favorite fruits overnight. Here are some creative options to try:

Juice Ice Cubes: Freeze your homemade juice into ice cubes for a refreshing twist.

Lemon and Lime Slices: Not only do they add zing, but they're also great for your liver and packed with Vitamin C.

Mint Leaves: Fresh and invigorating, mint aids digestion and adds a delightful fragrance.

Cinnamon Stick Infusion: Aids digestion increases blood circulation and helps stabilize blood sugar levels.

Ginger Slices: Known for improving digestion and reducing inflammation, ginger is a game-changer.

Basil Leaves: An excellent anti-inflammatory, basil leaves add a subtle yet distinct flavor.

Mix and match these recommendations to create your signature-infused water. One of my favorites is a blend of mint leaves, ginger, and lemon, and this can be acidic to some individuals and cause stomach discomfort, so proceed with caution to determine how your body processes these steps. For a fruity twist, try adding slices of strawberries, raspberries, and blackberries with a touch of mint.

Bonus Option: Soda Splash

If you are craving something fizzy, opt for sparkling or carbonated water; you may add lemon or lime slices. It's a guilt-free way to add sparkle to your hydration routine. With these creative steps, you will discover a world of refreshing flavors. It is all about finding what tickles your taste buds and nourishes your body.

Cold vs Hot vs Lukewarm Water: Lukewarm water wins because it is gentler and better for the skin. Of course, there are exemptions to this rule "One Size Does Not Fit All."

7 Strategies to Optimize Your Health & Prevent Chronic Illnesses.

Disclaimer: The following statistics are generalized and for reference only. Please note that these numbers are approximate based on an average adult human; some individual's organs may weigh slightly less or slightly more. Also, these numbers may be affected by age, sex, and nutrition/health status.

The Weight of Vital Organs: Male Body Organs

The human body is a marvelous design, and within it lies vital organs, each with its unique weight and significance. While these weights can vary based on many factors, here is a general overview of the average weights of major organs in an adult male.

Brain: 3 pounds

The brain, which weighs a remarkable three pounds, is the epicenter of intelligence and cognition. It orchestrates our thoughts, emotions, and movements, making it the command center of our existence.

Heart: 1 pound

The tireless champion of circulation, the heart weighs approximately one pound. With each beat, it pumps life-sustaining blood throughout our body, ensuring every cell receives the oxygen and nutrients it craves.

Kidneys: 2 pounds

The silent heroes of detoxification, the kidneys, come in at a combined weight of two pounds. They tirelessly filter waste and regulate our body's fluid and electrolyte balance.

Liver: 3 pounds

The liver, weighing three pounds, is the body's metabolic powerhouse. It processes nutrients, detoxifies harmful substances, and plays a pivotal role in digestion.

Lungs: 2 pounds

The breath of life, our lungs, collectively weigh approximately two pounds. They provide our cells with life-sustaining oxygen while expelling carbon dioxide, ensuring our bodies function optimally.

Pancreas: 6 ounces

The pancreas weighs six ounces, and it is a small yet mighty organ. It produces essential enzymes and hormones that aid digestion and regulate blood sugar levels.

Stomach: 2 pounds

The gateway to digestion, the stomach carries a weight of about two pounds. Its muscular walls swirl and break down food, preparing it for further processing in the intestines.

Intestines: 5 pounds

The network of the intestines tips the scales at approximately five pounds. They absorb nutrients and water from our food.

Spleen: 6 ounces

Though small, the spleen's importance is immeasurable. Weighing in at a mere six ounces, it aids in immune function and acts as a reservoir for blood, removing damaged and old blood cells and controlling red blood cells, white blood cells, and platelets. It contains white blood cells to fight germs in the bloodstream.

Gallbladder: 3 ounces

The gallbladder, a gallant companion to the liver, weighs a mere three ounces. It stores bile produced by the liver and releases it to aid in digestion as needed, and it helps break down fats.

Bladder: 1 pound

The reservoir for waste, the bladder, carries a weight of approximately one pound. It holds and releases urine, a vital process in our body's waste elimination.

While these average weights provide a fascinating glimpse into the internal workings of the human body, it is important to note that individual variations are beyond doubt. Your organ weights may differ based on a multitude of factors. The weight of these organs is not the sole determinant of your health. Regular check-ups and discussions with your healthcare professional offer the most accurate assessment.

7 Strategies to Optimize Your Health & Prevent Chronic Illnesses.

The Weight of Vital Organs: A Closer Look at the Female Body

The weight of major body organs is a subject that embraces diversity, influenced by a range of factors such as age, sex, height, weight, and body composition. The average weights of key organs in an adult female, acknowledging that individual variations are to be expected. These organs' main functionalities are kin to the male functions.

- Brain: Approximately 2.7 pounds
- Heart: Around 1 pound
- Kidneys: About 2 pounds
- Liver: Approximately 3 pounds
- Lungs: Roughly 2 pounds
- Pancreas: 6 ounces
- Stomach: About 2 pounds
- Intestines: Around 5 pounds
- Spleen: 6 ounces
- Gallbladder: 3 ounces
- Bladder: Approximately 1 pound

Factors Influencing Organ Weight: It is important to note that these figures are averages. The actual weight of an individual's organs may deviate based on a combination of factors, including age, sex, height, and body composition. This diversity is unique to everyone.

Organ Weight and Health: Weight alone does not serve as a definitive indicator of one's health. For example, an individual with a larger liver may still be in excellent health, while someone with a smaller liver may face liver-related health challenges.

Understanding the varying weights of major organs in the female body provides valuable insight into human physiology. It reminds us that health is a multifaceted concept encompassing various factors beyond organ weight. Consulting with a healthcare provider remains the most reliable method for evaluating one's health status.

Balancing the Scales: Understanding Total Body Fat

Total body fat is a critical component of our body's composition, playing a role in various physiological functions. Understanding its distribution and ideal percentages is vital.

Average Total Fat Weight: The average total fat weight in the United States differs slightly between adult males and females. For adult males, it is approximately 43.5 pounds, accounting for around 22% of their body weight. Adult females, on the other hand, have an average total fat weight of about 39.2 pounds, constituting roughly 25% of their body weight.

Variability and Factors: These figures are averages, and total fat weight varies based on several factors. Age, sex, height, weight, and overall body composition contribute to this variation; this highlights the individuality of body composition and the need for personalized health assessments.

Percentage versus Weight While total fat weight is significant, the percentage of total body fat holds even greater importance. This percentage reflects the proportion of fat mass to total body mass and provides a more accurate measure of individual overall weight and fat percentage weight. Do not focus on the overall weight you see on your scale since the fat percentage is a more accurate way to measure your excess weight and overall health.

Healthy Percentage Ranges A healthy percentage of total body fat for adult males typically falls between 15% and 20%. With their unique physiological requirements, adult females tend to have a healthy range between 20% and 25% total fat.

Seeking Professional Guidance: If you have concerns about your total body fat composition, consult a healthcare provider. They can provide personalized advice and assessments to help you understand your unique body composition and make informed health decisions.

Total body fat is a dynamic aspect of our physiological makeup, influencing various aspects of health. Recognizing the significance of both total fat weight and percentage allows individuals to take proactive steps toward achieving and maintaining body health.

The Vital Role of Muscle Mass in Human Physiology: Muscle mass constitutes a significant portion of our body's composition, impacting various aspects of our physical well-being. Human muscles comprise approximately 37-40% of total body weight; this means that for a person weighing 150 pounds, about 55-60 pounds is attributed to muscle mass.

Factors Influencing Muscle Mass: Muscle mass can vary significantly based on age, sex, height, weight, and overall body composition. For instance, men tend to possess higher muscle mass than women. Additionally, individuals who engage in regular physical activity tend to have greater muscle mass than those who lead a more sedentary lifestyle.

Importance of Muscle Mass: Muscle mass serves many crucial functions within the body. It is instrumental in maintaining strength, power, and balance, contributing significantly to physical performance. Moreover, muscles act as protective buffers for bones and joints, safeguarding against potential injuries. Additionally, muscle mass plays a pivotal role in metabolism, influencing energy expenditure and helping to regulate body weight. Muscle mass is a fundamental component of our physiological makeup, profoundly impacting our physical capabilities and health. Recognizing its significance encourages individuals to engage in activities that promote its development and maintenance.

Personalized Assessment and Planning: Conferring a healthcare provider or personal trainer is advisable if you have concerns regarding your muscle mass. They can conduct assessments for your specific circumstances and guide you on enhancing or sustaining your muscle mass effectively.

The Structural Significance of Bone Mass in Human Physiology: Bone mass constitutes a crucial element of our body's framework, offering support, protection, and other vital functions. Understanding its proportion and role is essential for comprehending your unique physical needs.

Average Bone Mass Percentage: Human bones account for approximately 14% of total body weight. For instance, in a person weighing 150 pounds, approximately 21 pounds are attributed to bone mass.

Factors Influencing Bone Mass: The actual quantity of bone mass can vary substantially based on age, sex, height, weight, and overall body composition. For instance, men tend to possess higher bone mass than women. Furthermore, bone mass tends to decrease with age, making older individuals have less bone mass than younger counterparts.

Significance of Bone Mass: Bone mass serves a multitude of vital roles within the body. It provides structural support to the body, forming a protective framework around internal organs. Moreover, bones are pivotal in producing red blood cells, essential for oxygen transportation. Additionally, bone mass contributes to metabolism, influences energy expenditure, and helps regulate body weight.

Maintaining Bone Health: Ensuring the health of your bones is crucial. Engaging in weight-bearing exercises, consuming a balanced diet rich in calcium and vitamin D, and avoiding smoking and excessive alcohol consumption are all important steps in maintaining bone health.

Bone mass is a critical component of our anatomical structure, significantly impacting our physical integrity and overall health. Recognizing its importance underscores the need for individuals to adopt lifestyle choices that promote bone health.

Journaling time

Think about how you can put the knowledge from this chapter into action in your daily life. How can you make it work for you?

_____
_____
_____
_____
_____
_____
_____
_____

"Those who think they have no time for healthy eating, will sooner or later have time for illness"- Edward Stanley

Chapter 5

Nutrition

Learning Objectives

- Balanced Nutrition vs diet plans
- Organic vs non-organic
- Non-GMO vs GMO
- What's the fuzz with the pesticides?
- Important Food Groups for optimal health
- Water
- Proteins
- Vitamins
- Minerals
- Carbohydrates
- Fats
- Dietary Fiber
- Sugar: An Enemy or A Friend
- Calories: The Good, Bad, and Ugly.
- Why Fruit & Vegetables are your best friends.
- Fat: Healthy vs Unhealthy
- Carbs: Good vs Bad guys. Starch:
- Protein: Life building Block
- Supplements: Do They Actually Work?
- Supplementation vs Natural Foods
- Food servings and recommendations
- Why does your BMI and weight not matter anymore?

- Listening to your Body: Why, When, what, How, and Where to eat
- Hunger Rating
- Satiation Rating
- 21 Days Meal Prep
- Freezing/Thawing foods
- Recipes
- Poop
- Body Taxation (BTT)
- Reading Food Labels
- Choices and Dark Side of Marketing (CDM)
- Importance of Balanced Nutrition for your body systems

A Revolutionary Approach to Health and Nutrition

This book is not about counting calories or stepping on the scale daily. Instead, it is about empowering you with the knowledge to make informed choices about the products you consume, steering clear of deceptive labels that claim to be "healthy." Brace yourself because you will redefine your relationship with food and nutrition.

A New Perspective on Nutrition: You will uncover a blueprint to help you make healthier choices and liberate yourself from the cycle of fad diets that often prove unsustainable in the long run. The goal is to equip you with the tools to prioritize your nutrition and establish boundaries with indulgent foods. It is time to break free from the constraints of conventional dieting.

Honesty and Self-Reflection: The backbone of this journey is honesty, not just with the world, but most importantly, with yourself. You are your most significant ally in this endeavor. Committing to giving your all and pushing beyond your limits will guarantee success and set the stage for a profound transformation. Promise yourself that you are not merely going to give 100% but are willing to go above and beyond. This is your commitment, and it is a promise worth keeping. With an open mind and immense dedication to your health, you are self-assured to begin a path that leads to a version of you that makes the best nutritional choices to nourish the universe within you. Are you ready?

Balanced Nutrition vs Diet Plans

The Foundation of Health: Balanced Nutrition
According to the Merriam-Webster Dictionary, *nutrition* is the act or process of nourishing or being nourished. Essentially, nutrition is the lifeline that sustains the organs and cells within our bodies, enabling them to function optimally. Achieving a balanced and wholesome diet is not just a matter of personal preference but a fundamental human survival requirement.

The Significance of Balanced Nutrition: Balanced nutrition is not merely an option but a prerequisite for overall health. It catalyzes a robust mind and body, protecting against many diseases. The impact of balanced nutrition is far-reaching, from safeguarding the brain, heart, and lungs to fortifying the gastrointestinal, renal, reproductive, and nervous systems. The benefits cascade across each body cell aimed to work properly.

Prevention Through Nourishment: The power of nutrition lies in its preventive capabilities. We can shield ourselves from many avoidable diseases by adopting a balanced diet. While the list of potential ailments is extensive, it suffices to say that balanced nutrition is a formidable defense against many health challenges.

Productivity and Well-being: Individuals who prioritize balanced nutrition not only enjoy heightened productivity but also experience a greater sense of fulfillment. Their lives are marked by vitality, happiness, and an optimistic outlook. Through the simple act of nourishing their bodies effectively, they can live longer, more vibrant lives.

In essence, nutrition is the foundation of a thriving existence. It is not just about satisfying hunger but about providing the body with the essential elements it needs to flourish. By embracing balanced nutrition, we fortify our physical health and cultivate a robust foundation for mental and emotional well-being. It is time to recognize the profound impact that our dietary choices have on the quality and longevity of our lives, leading to strong body cells, stronger organs, stronger and healthier body.

Balanced nutrition is when you eat/drink foods containing good sources of:
1- Water
2- Proteins
3- Fruits
4- Vegetables
5- Nutritious Fats
6- Natural Vitamins whenever possible.
7- Fiber-rich produce.
8- Minerals
9- Organic Dairy if not intolerant.
10- Whole Grain

Decoding Diets: The Maze of Diet Plans
At its core, a diet has become synonymous with a well-intentioned yet often ineffective long-term weight loss endeavor. However, the etymology of the term reveals a more profound meaning. Derived from the Greek word "diaita," diet originally referred to a "way of living." In the modern context, it has evolved into cycles that promise rapid weight loss yet frequently leave individuals disheartened and often heavier than when they began.

Modern Diets: In today's world, a staggering array of diets and eating plans exist, each touting its own set of benefits and restrictions. With over 100 distinct diets and more than 1,000 eating plans, the choices can be overwhelming. Many of these diets revolve around limiting or even completely excluding specific food groups in a bid to cut down on calorie intake. It is imperative to shed light on some of the most widely recognized approaches to navigate this labyrinth of dietary options.

The Pitfalls of Short-Term Thinking: While these diets often promise immediate results, they catch up in the long run. Their restrictive nature can lead to unsustainable practices and, in some cases, nutrient deficiencies. The cycle of deprivation followed by indulgence perpetuates a frustrating cycle, ultimately hindering the pursuit of sustainable, balanced nutrition. We must approach diets with discernment in our quest for optimal health. Understanding that proper nourishment extends beyond short-lived regimens empowers us to seek sustainable, balanced approaches to eating. Rather than being confined by the limitations of diets, we can embrace a holistic "way of living."

Before you continue, I am curious about your thoughts about diets, your experiences with them, and how they make you feel.

_____

_____

_____

_____

Exploring Dietary Philosophies: In today's diverse world, dietary choices have transcended mere sustenance to become profound statements about our values, ethics, and health concerns. They also discuss various dietary philosophies, shedding light on the principles that guide their practitioners. Dietary choices have evolved into multifaceted expressions of our values, beliefs, and health aspirations. Each philosophy carries ethical and health considerations, urging us to reflect on our place within the intricate web of human and environmental well-being.

Characteristics of a Plant-Based Diet (Vegan): A plant-based diet, commonly known as a vegan diet, is a dietary approach that exclusively includes foods derived from plants.

Fruits and Vegetables: These form the foundation of a plant-based diet. Emphasis is placed on various colorful fruits and vegetables, which provide essential vitamins, minerals, fiber, and antioxidants.

Green Leafy Vegetables are particularly encouraged due to their high nutrient density. They are rich in vitamins, minerals, and phytochemicals that support optimal health.

Whole Grains: This includes brown rice, quinoa, whole wheat bread, and oats. Whole grains are a significant source of complex carbohydrates, fiber, and essential nutrients.

Legumes: This category encompasses beans, lentils, chickpeas, and other plant-based protein sources. Legumes are high in protein, fiber, and various vitamins and minerals.

Nuts and Seeds: These are excellent sources of healthy fats, protein, and various nutrients. Examples include almonds, walnuts, chia seeds, flaxseeds, and hemp seeds.

Tofu and Plant-Based Protein Alternatives: Tofu, tempeh, and seitan are popular plant-based protein sources. Additionally, many meat substitutes are available that are made from plant-based ingredients like soy, mushrooms, or legumes.

Exclusion of Animal Products: Vegans abstain from all animal products, including meat, fish, dairy, eggs, and honey. This extends to non-food products derived from animals, such as leather, silk, and wool.

Avoidance of Animal-Tested Cosmetics and Products: Ethical vegans also refrain from using cosmetics, toiletries, and other products that have been tested on animals.

Plant-Based Diet: Health Benefits

Reduced risk of chronic diseases: Plant-based diets have been associated with lower rates of heart disease, high blood pressure, certain cancers, and type 2 diabetes.

Weight management: A well-balanced plant-based diet can support healthy weight loss or maintenance due to its lower calorie density and high fiber content.

Improved digestion: Plant-based foods' high fiber content aids digestion and helps prevent conditions like constipation.

Environmental Impact: Reduced carbon footprint: Plant-based diets typically have a lower environmental impact in terms of greenhouse gas emissions, land use, and water consumption compared to animal-based diets.

Ethical Considerations: Animal welfare: Many people adopt a vegan lifestyle out of ethical concerns for animal welfare, aiming to minimize harm to animals and promote compassionate living.

Support for a Sustainable Food System: Plant-based agriculture tends to be more efficient regarding land and water use, making it a potentially more sustainable option for feeding a growing global population.

Promotion of Culinary Diversity: Plant-based diets encourage exploration and creativity in the kitchen, as they offer a wide range of flavors, textures, and cooking techniques. Individuals following a plant-based diet must ensure they meet their nutritional needs, particularly for nutrients like vitamin B12, vitamin D, omega-3 fatty acids, iron, and calcium. Consulting a health coach, holistic registered dietitian, or healthcare provider can help create a well-balanced and nutritionally adequate plant-based eating plan.

The Mediterranean Diet: A Wholesome Approach to Health and Longevity

The Mediterranean Diet is a dietary pattern inspired by the traditional eating habits of countries bordering the Mediterranean Sea. It is renowned for emphasizing whole, minimally processed foods and has been linked to numerous health benefits.

Key Components of the Mediterranean Diet

Abundance of Fruits and Vegetables: These form the foundation of the Mediterranean Diet. They are rich in vitamins, minerals, antioxidants, and dietary fiber.

Emphasis on Whole Grains: Whole grains like brown rice, quinoa, whole wheat bread, and oats are preferred over refined grains. They provide complex carbohydrates, fiber, and essential nutrients.

Healthy Fats from Olive Oil: Olive oil is a primary source of fat in the Mediterranean Diet. It is rich in monounsaturated fats, which have been associated with heart health.

Legumes: Beans, lentils, and chickpeas are common sources of protein and fiber in Mediterranean cuisine. They are versatile ingredients in soups, stews, salads, and side dishes.

Nuts and Seeds: Moderately consumed almonds, walnuts, chia seeds, flaxseeds, and other nuts and seeds provide healthy fats, protein, and various nutrients.

Seafood and Lean Proteins: Fish, particularly fatty fish like salmon, mackerel, and sardines, are central to the Mediterranean Diet. Poultry, eggs, and dairy products are also included in moderation.

Limited Red Meat Consumption: Red meat is consumed infrequently in the Mediterranean Diet. When it is consumed, it is often in small quantities and as part of mixed dishes.

Moderate Dairy Intake: Greek yogurt, cheese, and other dairy products are enjoyed in moderation and provide calcium and protein.

Minimal Processed Foods: The Mediterranean Diet encourages whole, minimally processed foods and discourages the consumption of highly processed and refined products.

Herbs and Spices: Fresh herbs and spices are used liberally to flavor dishes, reducing the need for excessive salt and unhealthy condiments.

Additional Characteristics: In some versions of the Mediterranean Diet, moderate red wine consumption with meals is included. However, this is optional and should be done in moderation.

Health Benefits of the Mediterranean Diet

Heart Health: The Mediterranean Diet has been associated with a reduced risk of heart disease. Combining healthy fats, fiber-rich foods, and antioxidants supports heart health.

Weight Management: The diet's focus on whole, nutrient-dense foods can contribute to healthy weight management.

Improved Cognitive Function: Some studies suggest that the Mediterranean Diet may support cognitive function and reduce the risk of cognitive decline.

Reduced Inflammation: The abundance of anti-inflammatory foods in this diet may help reduce chronic inflammation, which is linked to many chronic diseases such as Alzheimer's disease, type 2 diabetes, asthma, cancer, heart disease, and Rheumatoid Arthritis. Inflammation can lead to abdominal pain, joint pain, fatigue, and skin issues, among many other ailments.

Better Blood Sugar Control: The Mediterranean Diet may be beneficial for individuals with type 2 diabetes or those at risk of developing it.

Longevity: Some research suggests that adherence to the Mediterranean Diet is associated with a longer lifespan and reduced mortality rates.

The Mediterranean Diet offers a balanced and sustainable approach to healthy eating. It encourages a variety of nutrient-rich foods and can be adapted to individual preferences and cultural practices.

The Vegetarian Diet: Nourishing the Body, Mind, and Planet

The vegetarian diet focuses on plant-based foods while excluding meat, fish, and poultry. It is a nutritionally balanced approach that emphasizes fruits, vegetables, whole grains, nuts, seeds, legumes, dairy products, and eggs. This diet is renowned for its numerous health benefits, positive environmental impact, and ethical considerations.

Plant-Based Emphasis: One of the core principles of the vegetarian diet is the abundance of plant-based foods. This includes various colorful fruits and vegetables rich in essential vitamins, minerals, antioxidants, and fiber.

Nutritional Balance: Vegetarians have various options to ensure they meet their nutritional needs. Protein sources like beans, lentils, tofu, tempeh, and dairy products provide ample protein. Whole grains such as quinoa, brown rice, and whole wheat bread offer complex carbohydrates, while nuts and seeds deliver healthy fats. A well-planned vegetarian diet can provide all the nutrients for a healthy lifestyle.

Exclusion of Animal Products: Vegetarians abstain from consuming animals, which means they do not include meat, fish, and poultry in their diets. This choice is often made for various reasons, including ethical concerns, animal welfare, and personal beliefs.

Health Benefits: Studies have consistently shown that well-balanced vegetarian diets are associated with numerous health benefits. These include a reduced risk of heart disease, lower blood pressure, improved cholesterol levels, and better blood sugar control. Additionally, vegetarians often have lower rates of obesity and certain types of cancer.

Environmental Impact: The vegetarian diet has a significantly lower environmental footprint than diets that include meat. Livestock farming significantly contributes to greenhouse gas emissions, deforestation, and water pollution. By choosing plant-based options, individuals contribute to a more sustainable and eco-friendly food system.

Ethical Considerations: For many vegetarians, their dietary choice is motivated by ethical concerns regarding the treatment of animals. They believe in promoting a compassionate lifestyle by avoiding products that harm or exploit animals.

Variety and Creativity: The vegetarian diet encourages culinary creativity and exploration. Countless delicious and nutritious recipes are available with an extensive array of plant-based ingredients. From hearty bean stews to vibrant vegetable stir-fries, the possibilities are endless.

Considerations for a Balanced Diet: While a vegetarian diet offers numerous benefits, it is important to ensure it is well-balanced. This includes incorporating various plant-based protein sources, consuming fortified foods or supplements for nutrients like vitamin B12 and paying attention to iron and calcium intake. In conclusion, the vegetarian diet is a holistic approach to nutrition that offers many benefits for individuals and the planet. By embracing a diet centered around plant-based foods, individuals can promote their health, contribute to environmental sustainability, and align with ethical values. A vegetarian diet can be enjoyable and nourishing with careful planning and a diverse selection of plant foods.

Pescatarians: Environmental and Health Considerations

Pescatarian is a dietary choice that threads the needle between vegetarianism and a broader omnivorous approach. It allows for a diet rich in plant-based foods, including fish, shellfish, and select animal-derived products. Beyond its health benefits, pescatarians pose an environmentally conscious option, although it necessitates a nuanced understanding of the potential risks of seafood consumption.

Environmental Consciousness: Pescatarians often address environmental concerns. Opting for fish and seafood as protein sources can alleviate the environmental impact of large-scale livestock farming. However, one must tread with awareness, considering the broader implications of fish farming. This type of farming can be unethical and cause serious health issues.

Mercury Toxicity and Microplastic Concerns: While seafood is a valuable source of essential nutrients, it is crucial to acknowledge the potential risks. High consumption of certain fish and shellfish can lead to mercury toxicity, presenting a spectrum of symptoms ranging from mild cognitive effects to severe physical impairments. Additionally, microplastics, stemming from the breakdown of plastics in marine environments, pose a growing concern. They infiltrate sea creatures' tissues and eventually enter the human diet.

The Complex World of Fish Farming: The practice of fish farming, though aimed at meeting the rising demand for seafood, introduces its challenges. Crowded conditions and suboptimal feed quality can lead to health issues among farmed fish. This often necessitates antibiotics and vaccinations, further highlighting the complexities associated with this approach. Not to mention the poor-quality foods fed to farm-raised seafood, unethical farmers will feed these creatures foods that are not even part of their food chain; this alters their DNA and causes health issues when humans eat the unethical-raised seafood.

Prioritizing Wild-Caught Seafood: Choosing wild-caught seafood over farmed options comes with a higher price tag, but it is a conscious investment in personal health and ethical seafood sourcing. Wild-caught seafood offers a more natural and balanced nutritional profile while promoting sustainable fishing practices. In conclusion, pescatarians represent a balanced dietary choice, merging the benefits of plant-based nutrition with including seafood. However, it demands a thorough understanding of environmental and health considerations. By navigating potential risks and making informed choices, individuals can embrace pescatarians as a conscientious approach to personal well-being and environmental sustainability.

Paleolithic Diet: Ancient Wisdom or Modern Misconception?

The Paleolithic diet, popularly known as the Paleo diet, traces its roots back to the pioneering work of gastroenterologist Walter Voegtlin in the 1970s. Voegtlin's premise was intriguing: By emulating the dietary patterns of our Paleolithic ancestors, we could potentially mitigate a range of gastrointestinal issues, including indigestion, diabetes, and obesity. While the diet allows for certain foods like grass-fed meats, fish, plant-based fare, and nuts, it rigidly excludes processed flour and dairy and emphasizes honey as the primary sweetener. Nevertheless, the diet's efficacy and long-term implications remain a subject of vigorous debate.

The Paleo Paradigm: The heart of the Paleo diet lies in its commitment to whole, unprocessed foods. Advocates argue that this approach mirrors the dietary habits of our ancient forebears, potentially offering a more natural and nutrient-dense alternative to modern eating patterns.

The Exclusionary Principle: Processed foods, salt, and dairy bear the brunt of the Paleo diet's prohibitions. This stems from the belief that our ancestors subsisted on minimally processed fare, free from the additives and preservatives that typify contemporary diets. By avoiding these elements, proponents assert that we can reduce inflammation and enhance overall health.

Unearthing Controversy: Critics, however, raise a chorus of concerns. Studies examining ancient mummies have uncovered signs of hardened arteries, challenging the notion that our ancestors were free from heart disease. Moreover, life expectancy in the Paleolithic era was markedly lower than today, casting doubt on the diet's suitability for modern, longer-lived humans.

Balancing the Scales: The Paleo diet prompts important questions about the potential benefits of returning to a more 'ancestral' way of eating. However, it also underscores the complexities of drawing direct dietary comparisons across millennia. As researchers continue to unravel the mysteries of human nutrition, a balanced approach that incorporates both ancestral wisdom and contemporary scientific understanding may hold the key to optimal health. In conclusion, the Paleo diet has potential implications for modern nutrition. While it invites us to reconsider our dietary choices, it also challenges us to evaluate human health's complexities across the ages critically. Balancing the lessons left by our ancestors in history with the present insights, we can forge a path toward nourishment that honors our ancient heritage and our present-day needs.

Detox Diets: Dilemma & Controversy

Detox diets have ignited a typhoon of debate within the world of nutrition. Advocates claim they offer a respite from synthetic chemicals and heavy metals that pervade our daily lives, while skeptics question their effectiveness and potential health risks. Navigating this terrain requires a discerning eye, as financial interests often shape the narrative. Amidst the controversy, a critical question emerges: can a well-executed detox pave the way for lasting health benefits, or does it merely offer a short-lived spare?

The Toxic Truth: In an era inundated with processed and fast foods, our bodies contend with a steady influx of toxins (free radicals). These substances, originating from the products we consume, the air we breathe, and the items we use, accumulate over time, potentially leading to various diseases and ailments.

Unearthing the Detox Diet: Detox diets emerge as a potential remedy, promising to purge the body of accumulated toxins and even facilitate weight loss. They typically incorporate foods and practices known for their detoxifying properties, ranging from teas and supplements to juicing and water pills.

The Short-Term Solution Dilemma: A recurring challenge with detox diets lies in their transience. Many individuals embrace these diets briefly, only to revert to former habits once the detox period concludes. This cycle raises questions about the sustainability and long-term efficacy of such approaches.

A Lifetime of Detoxification: A glimmer of hope arises when detoxification is approached judiciously and with a long-term perspective. When executed health-consciously, a detox regimen can catalyze enduring change, instilling healthier habits that withstand the test of time. In conclusion, the detox diet, a subject of fervent discussion, embodies promise and peril. While its effectiveness and safety remain contested, the question remains: Can a detox pave the way for a healthier, toxin-free existence?

The Nordic Diet: A Collage of Wellness

Hailing from the rich culinary traditions of Scandinavia, the Nordic Diet presents a time-honored approach to nutrition. Centered around wild-caught seafood, locally sourced produce, and a touch of canola oil, this diet mirrors the revered Mediterranean regimen, even with a distinctly Nordic flair. Beyond its gustatory delights, the Nordic Diet unveils a treasured aggregation of health benefits, ranging from cholesterol management to cancer risk reduction. The foundation of the Nordic Diet lies in its emphasis on wild seafood, a tribute to the pristine waters that grace the region. This diet is adorned with an array of earthy root vegetables, including beets, carrots, and turnips, which add depth to its flavor profile and offer a host of nutritional rewards.

Whole Grains: The Nordic Foundation: The humble yet nutritionally potent whole grains, such as oats, barley, and rye, are anchoring this diet. These grains serve as companions in the quest for optimal health and vitality.

From Sea to Plate: The Seafood Symphony: Tuna, wild salmon, mackerel, and sardines form the seafood ensemble of the Nordic Diet. While their taste and aroma may evoke unique sensations, their health benefits far outweigh culinary reservations.

Legumes and Low-Fat Dairy: This diet adds legumes and low-fat dairy options, providing a well-rounded nutritional profile that caters to both satiety and vitality.

Eggs and Game Meat: A Prudent Indulgence: Eggs and game meats, such as rabbit, elk, and even alligator, are celebrated in moderation, offering a distinctive twist to the Nordic palate.

Steering Clear: Dietary No-Nos: While the Nordic Diet celebrates many wholesome options, it sternly shuns a few dietary culprits. Alcoholic beverages, non-game meats, processed meats, high-sodium fare, sugary indulgences, and fast foods find no sanctuary within this regimen.

In conclusion, the Nordic Diet is steeped in tradition and brimming with nutritional wisdom. With each plate, we savor the flavors of the north and partake in healthful benefits that resonate throughout our bodies.

Intermittent Fasting: A Time-Centric Approach to Wellness

Intermittent fasting is a nutritional paradigm that hinges on designated periods of nourishment followed by deliberate fasting intervals with unique strategies for optimizing health. While diverse methodologies exist, a safer approach – a structured eating window according to your body's needs. Some people fast for eight hours, others can safely fast for twelve hours, and others can be harmonized by a disciplined 16-hour fasting period or longer. Consult with your primary healthcare professional before starting any intermittent fasting approach if you have any chronic health issues.

Intermittent Fasting Demystified: The essence of intermittent fasting lies in its time-bound approach. By adhering to this regimen, we grant our bodies a respite from constant digestion, allowing them to recalibrate and rejuvenate during fasting.

The Eight-Hour Feast: During the eight-hour feeding window, nourishing our bodies with wholesome, balanced meals takes precedence. This period serves as an opportunity to partake in a medley of nutrient-dense foods that fuel and fortify.

The Sixteen-Hour Sanctuary: The fasting phase, spanning 16 hours, signals the body to a state of rest. During this period, metabolic pathways shift, paving the way for autophagy, cellular rejuvenation, and ketosis, using stored fat for energy.

Listening to Your Body: In the intermittent fasting world, attentiveness to bodily cues is imperative. Should discomfort or distress arise, it is important to honor these signals and adjust the fasting duration accordingly. Please pay attention to your body's cues when it is time to break the fasting. For example, increased weakness, dehydration, headaches, increased fatigue, irritability, difficulty concentrating, fainting, increased respirations, extreme hunger, extreme weight loss, low blood pressure symptoms (dizziness, lightheadedness, sleepiness, weakness, fainting, confusion, blurred vision, nausea, or vomiting).

The Varied Faces of Intermittent Fasting: While our focus is primarily on the eight-hour feeding window and 16-hour fasting, it is crucial to acknowledge the diverse approaches to intermittent fasting. Some methodologies, while promising, may carry potential risks, underscoring the importance of prudent discernment. In conclusion, with its structured interplay between nourishment, intermittent fasting extends an invitation to a harmonious relationship with our bodies. Pay close attention to your body's cues.

The Low-Fat Enigma: Separating Fact from Fiction

Low-fat diets have long been a subject of discourse and debate on nutrition. While it seems to be a universal remedy for health, it is imperative to dissect the nuances of such dietary choices and understand their potential implications.

The Low-Fat Paradox: One of the perplexing aspects of low-fat diets lies in their propensity to elevate carbohydrate intake. This shift can culminate in heightened levels of triglycerides, a type of fat in the blood, potentially predisposing individuals to cardiovascular diseases.

Deciphering the Dynamics of Low-Carb Diets: Weight Loss and Beyond

Many people find low-fat diets confusing because they often consume more carbohydrates to compensate for the reduction in fat. However, this change in dietary habits can result in elevated triglyceride levels, fats found in the bloodstream. When these levels are high, it can increase the risk of developing cardiovascular diseases. Some studies have shown that a high-carbohydrate diet can be more detrimental to heart health than a diet high in fat. Therefore, it is important to be mindful of the types of carbohydrates you consume and aim for a balanced diet that includes healthy fats, protein, and complex carbohydrates.

Low Carb, High Impact: Low-carb diets are renowned for their efficacy in facilitating rapid weight loss. However, it is imperative to acknowledge that sustaining this weight loss presents a considerable challenge for many individuals. One notable benefit of low-carb diets is their capacity to regulate triglyceride levels. Triglycerides, fatty molecules in the bloodstream, are pivotal in cardiovascular health. By curbing their excess, low-carb diets may offer a protective effect.

Nevertheless, overdoing it can cause issues as well. While low-carb diets can trigger initial weight loss, the long-term retention of this achievement remains a complex endeavor. The challenges are present in the diet and the sustainable lifestyle changes accompanying it.

Strategic Carbohydrate Selection: Rather than outright reduction, the emphasis in low-carb diets should be on the type of carbohydrates consumed. Prioritizing complex, fiber-rich sources over refined counterparts ensures sustained energy levels without dramatic blood sugar fluctuations. Refined carbohydrates are often called simple, refined, or bad carbs.

The Role of Protein: Regarding low-carb diets, protein is a fundamental component that plays a significant role in keeping you full and maintaining muscle mass. Achieving a balance between protein and other macronutrients is crucial for maximizing the advantages of a low-carb approach.

Beyond the Scale: Holistic Well-Being: While weight loss is a pivotal facet of low-carb diets, their impact extends beyond mere numbers on a scale. These diets can influence metabolic markers, insulin sensitivity, and cardiovascular health. However, their long-term viability hinges on prudent dietary choices, balanced macronutrient intake, and sustainable lifestyle modifications. In conclusion, individuals can make better-informed decisions by understanding low-carb nutrition.

The Carnivore Diet Approach: A Closer Look at the All-Meat Diet

The Carnivore diet, characterized by an exclusive reliance on animal products, has gained traction for its radical departure from conventional dietary norms. This dietary approach advocates the complete exclusion of carbohydrates, relying solely on consuming meat, fish, and eggs.

Meat-Heavy Metabolism: The unapologetic emphasis on animal-based foods is central to the Carnivore diet. Proponents argue that this dietary composition aligns with our ancestral roots, providing a nutrient-dense foundation.

Nutritional Density: Meat, an undisputed nutritional powerhouse, has essential proteins, vitamins, and minerals crucial for bodily functions.

However, excluding plant-based foods raises concerns about potential nutrient deficiencies, particularly in fiber, vitamins C and E, and various phytonutrients.

Inflammation and the Carnivore Connection: While proponents praise the Carnivore diet for its potential to alleviate certain inflammatory conditions, critics caution against the potential for heightened inflammation due to the exclusive reliance on animal products. Balancing the benefits with potential risks remains a pivotal consideration.

Addressing Ethical and Environmental Concerns: Beyond health implications, the Carnivore diet sparks ethical and environmental debates. The substantial reliance on animal agriculture raises questions about sustainability, animal welfare, and ecological impact.

The Quest for Long-Term Viability: Sustainability is a primary concern when evaluating the Carnivore diet's long-term viability. Striking a balance between reaping the potential benefits and mitigating potential risks necessitates meticulous planning and consideration.

Dietary Dissonance: While the Carnivore diet offers a distinctive approach to nutrition, its departure from conventional dietary norms calls for a critical examination of potential benefits and risks. Engaging in open dialogue and consulting with healthcare professionals can offer invaluable insights. In conclusion, the Carnivore diet dietary approaches are available today. While its unique composition may benefit some, a cautious evaluation of potential risks and long-term implications remains imperative. By weighing the merits against the concerns, you can make informed decisions about your nutritional journey.

The Crash Diet Conundrum: Quick Fixes, Lasting Impact?

Crash diets, characterized by their extreme calorie restriction and rapid weight loss goals, have become a prevalent approach for those seeking swift results. This dietary strategy hinges on drastically reducing food intake to levels that may only sustain essential bodily functions. At the core of crash diets lies a drastic reduction in caloric intake, often far below the recommended daily intake. This approach aims to force the body into a caloric deficit, potentially leading to rapid weight loss.

Metabolic Confusion: While crash diets may yield initial weight loss, severe caloric restriction can precipitate a host of metabolic adaptations. These include a slowdown in metabolism, loss of lean muscle mass, and changes in hormonal regulation, all of which can hinder long-term weight management. This metabolic confusion can increase the risk for metabolic syndrome. Metabolic syndrome is a mixture of illnesses that increases the risk of stroke, diabetes, and coronary heart disease. Individuals with obesity, low HDL cholesterol (good cholesterol), high blood pressure, and high blood sugar levels are at higher risk of developing metabolic syndrome.

Nutrient Deficiency Dilemma: The stringent restrictions inherent in crash diets can lead to a deficiency in essential nutrients. The exclusion of food groups or severely limited food variety may result in inadequate intake of vital vitamins, minerals, and macronutrients.

The Rebound Effect: Crash diets' drastic nature often leads to an unsustainable eating pattern. When normal eating resumes, individuals may experience a rebound effect, regaining lost weight and sometimes surpassing their initial starting weights.

Psychological Impact: Crash diets can exert a toll on one's mental and emotional well-being. The stress and rigidity associated with extreme dietary restrictions may lead to feelings of deprivation, frustration, and a strained relationship with food.

Longevity and Lifestyle Considerations: While crash diets may yield swift results, their suitability for long-term adherence and overall lifestyle integration remains dubious. Such a restricted eating approach poses challenges in maintaining a balanced, sustainable, and enjoyable dietary pattern. In conclusion, crash diets, though alluring in their promise of swift transformation, come with many potential risks and limitations. Prioritizing a balanced, sustainable approach to nutrition and seeking professional guidance can pave the way for long-lasting, healthier lifestyle choices.

The Fad Diet Folly: Short-Lived Solutions, Long-Term Challenges

Fad diets, a prevalent phenomenon in nutrition, often promise quick fixes and dramatic results. However, these dietary trends are characterized by their transitory nature, exclusion of entire food groups, and a lack of emphasis on sustainable lifestyle changes.

The Appeal of Fad Diets: Fad diets gain popularity for their alluring promise of rapid weight loss and simplicity. They often offer a clear-cut set of rules, providing structure and direction for individuals seeking dietary guidance.

The Exclusion Enigma: One of the defining features of fad diets is the exclusion of entire food groups, labeling them as 'good' or 'bad'. While this approach may yield initial results, it can lead to potential nutrient deficiencies and an unbalanced intake of essential vitamins, minerals, and macronutrients.

The Binge-Restrict Cycle: Deprivation, a key factor of many fad diets, can inadvertently trigger a cycle of deprivation and indulgence. Prohibiting certain foods may increase one's desire for them, potentially resulting in episodes of overconsumption.

Lack of Long-Term Sustainability: Fad diets, by nature, are not designed for long-term adherence. The strict rules and limited food choices can become challenging to maintain over extended periods, making it likely that individuals will revert to previous eating patterns.

The Importance of Individualization: Each person's dietary needs, preferences, and tolerances are unique. Fad diets often fail to account for this individual variability, potentially leading to an unsuitable approach that may not align with one's health and wellness goals.

The Role of Exercise: Many fad diets place minimal emphasis on physical activity, neglecting the critical role that regular exercise plays in overall health and well-being. An appropriate physical activity regimen should complement a balanced approach to nutrition.

Medical Diets

Medical diets are specialized plans to address specific health conditions or nutritional needs. Healthcare professionals curate these diets to optimize health outcomes for individuals facing various health challenges.

The Purpose of Medical Diets: Unlike fad diets, which often focus solely on weight loss, medical diets manage and mitigate health conditions. These diets aim to provide essential nutrients while minimizing factors that may exacerbate medical issues.

Examples of Medical Diets

Diabetic Diet: Aims to regulate blood sugar levels, the diabetic diet emphasizes complex carbohydrates, fiber-rich foods, lean proteins, and healthy fats. It plays a crucial role in managing diabetes and preventing complications.

Cardiac Diet: Strategically constructed to promote heart health, this diet reduces saturated fats, cholesterol, and sodium. It prioritizes whole grains, lean proteins, fruits, vegetables, and heart-healthy fats.

Lactose-Free Diet: Recommended for individuals with lactose intolerance, this diet excludes dairy products and incorporates lactose-free alternatives to prevent digestive discomfort.

Low Fat/Cholesterol Diet: Targeted at reducing cholesterol levels, this diet limits the intake of saturated and trans fats. It emphasizes foods that lower cholesterol, such as fruits, vegetables, whole grains, and lean proteins.

The Role of Healthcare Professionals: Medical diets require professional oversight. Health coaches, holistic registered dietitians or healthcare providers play a pivotal role in monitoring these diets to individual needs, monitoring progress, and making necessary adjustments.

Personalization is Key: Each medical diet is created to address the specific health concerns of the individual. Factors such as age, gender, activity level, and medical history are considered in crafting a suitable dietary plan.

Balancing Nutrient Intake: While medical diets are designed to address specific health conditions, they must also provide a balanced intake of essential nutrients. This guards against potential deficiencies.

Sustainability and Long-Term Health: The goal of medical diets is to foster long-term health and wellness. Education, support, and ongoing guidance from healthcare professionals are integral in maintaining the dietary changes necessary for sustained health benefits. In conclusion, medical diets are invaluable healthcare tools, offering nutrition to individuals facing specific health challenges. With the guidance of healthcare professionals, these diets enhance the quality of life and effectively manage health conditions.

Faith-Based Diets: Nourishment in Accordance with Religious Principles

Religion profoundly influences many aspects of life, including dietary practices. Faith-based diets, rooted in religious teachings and traditions, provide guidelines for acceptable and appropriate consumption. Two prominent examples are the Kosher diet in Judaism and the Halal diet in Islam.

Kosher Diet
Guiding Principles: The Kosher diet adheres to the dietary laws outlined in the Torah, the sacred text of Judaism. These laws, known as Kashrut, dictate what is considered "fit" or "proper" to eat.

Key Restrictions and Practices

Meat and Dairy Separation: One of the fundamental rules of Kashrut is the prohibition of mixing meat and dairy products. This extends to both the cooking process and the utensils used.

Waiting Period: Observers wait a designated period, usually one hour, after consuming meat before they can partake in dairy products. Eggs, considered "pareve," are an exception.

Dish Differentiation: Specific dishes and utensils designated for meat or dairy preparation and consumption.

Prohibited Foods: Pork and shellfish are strictly prohibited in a Kosher diet.

Islam Diet (Halal)

Guiding Principles: Halal, meaning "lawful" or "permissible" in Arabic, refers to foods that align with Islamic dietary laws as detailed in the Quran.

Key Restrictions and Practices

Prohibition of Pork: Pork and its by-products are strictly forbidden in Islamic dietary practices.

Slaughter Method: Animals must be slaughtered in the name of Allah by a trained Muslim individual. This practice is known as Zabiha or Dhabihah.

Avoidance of Intoxicants: Alcohol and any intoxicating substances are considered Haram (forbidden).

Halal Certification: Many food products are labeled as Halal-certified to ensure they meet the dietary requirements.

Shared Values

Emphasis on Cleanliness: Kosher and Halal diets emphasize cleanliness and the avoidance of impurities in food preparation and consumption.

Respect for Life: Kosher and Halal dietary practices are rooted in a strong commitment to animal welfare and maintaining high standards of cleanliness in food preparation and consumption. By adhering to these practices, individuals maintain a healthy and balanced lifestyle and contribute to a more compassionate and ethical food system.

Honoring Faith Through Nourishment: The Kosher and Halal diets demonstrate how religious beliefs can permeate everyday life, including the food we consume. Adhering to these dietary practices allows individuals to observe their religious convictions and maintain a sense of spiritual and physical well-being. In the case of Halal, sourcing food from animals that have been slaughtered in accordance with Islamic guidelines and the careful selection of dairy products ensures that every aspect of their diet aligns with their faith. This conscientious approach to nourishment strengthens the connection between one's religious beliefs and daily sustenance.

The Atkins Diet: Low-Carb Approach to Weight Management

The Atkins Diet, developed by Dr. Robert Atkins in the 1970s, gained popularity for its emphasis on reducing carbohydrate intake to induce weight loss. It operates on the premise that by limiting carbs, the body shifts from using glucose for energy to burning stored fat, known as ketosis. This transition often leads to significant initial weight loss, making it an attractive option for those seeking quick results. The diet is divided into phases. In the initial phase, Induction, carbohydrate intake is severely restricted to jumpstart ketosis. This phase is followed by phases where carb intake gradually increases, allowing for a more balanced approach to nutrition. The goal is to find a sustainable level of carbohydrate consumption that supports weight management without compromising health. While the Atkins Diet has seen success stories, it is important to acknowledge potential drawbacks. Some individuals need help to adhere to the strict carb limitations, leading to discontinuation. Additionally, critics argue that the emphasis on protein and fat sources can sometimes lead to excessive consumption of saturated fats. For some, particularly those with specific health concerns like diabetes or cardiovascular issues, modifications may be necessary.

Ultimately, the Atkins Diet, like many dietary approaches, is not a universal solution. When choosing a nutritional plan, individuals must consider their unique health goals, preferences, and any underlying medical conditions. Consulting with a health coach, holistic registered dietitian, or healthcare provider can create personalized guidance and ensure dietary changes align with individual health needs. Moreover, long-term studies on the diet's effects are still evolving, and there is ongoing debate within the medical community about its sustainability and impact on overall health. Remember, what works best for one person may not be the ideal solution for another.

The Mayo Clinic Diet: Tailored Menus for Every Lifestyle

The Mayo Clinic Diet stands out in the dieting world for its versatility and practicality. Instead of a one-size-fits-all approach, it provides six distinct menu options, each meticulously designed to cater to various lifestyles. Whether you are looking to up your protein intake, explore the benefits of a healthy Keto approach, embrace a vegetarian lifestyle, or savor the rich flavors of the Mediterranean, the Mayo Clinic Diet has you covered.

This approach empowers individuals to select a menu that aligns seamlessly with their unique preferences, dietary needs, and health goals.

The Keto Diet: A Brief History and Potential Pitfalls

Originating as an epilepsy treatment in 1924 by Dr. Russell Wilder at the Mayo Clinic, the Keto diet has garnered attention for its distinctive approach. Like many others, this diet is marked by its restrictive nature, emphasizing low carbohydrate intake and a higher consumption of fats. While it has shown promise in some instances, it is important to tread carefully.

Adopting a Keto lifestyle may lead to a variety of outcomes. Some individuals may experience gastrointestinal issues, fluctuations in cholesterol levels, and even flu-like symptoms called "Keto Flu" during the initial phase; it can last from seven to fourteen days, sometimes even longer. The premise behind Keto lies in utilizing stored fat as the primary source of fuel—a bit like dipping into your savings account for an immediate purchase rather than waiting for the next paycheck; this can yield initial weight loss, but it is crucial to be aware of potential plateaus and the risk of your body entering a state of conservation, ultimately leading to the retention of depleted fat stores, along with feelings of frustration and defeat. Balance and moderation are key in any dietary journey.

The World of WW Inc: "A Holistic Approach to Wellness"

Formerly known as Weight Watchers, now rebranded as WW Inc., this program has evolved, reflecting a dynamic approach to achieving overall well-being. At its core, WW emphasizes a multi-faceted approach to weight loss, encompassing not only dietary considerations but also hydration, fitness, sleep, and meditation.

One key feature of the WW approach is calorie counting. Rather than a one-size-fits-all system, each food and beverage is assigned specific point values, providing individuals with a framework for making dietary choices. This approach encourages a conscious and balanced approach to eating, allowing individuals to align their consumption with their unique goals and preferences.

As with any wellness journey, individual results may vary. By incorporating these elements into a daily routine, WW Inc. aims to empower individuals to take charge of their health.

Professional Guidance and Education: Before initiating any dietary regimen, seeking guidance from a qualified health coach, holistic registered dietitian, or healthcare provider is crucial. These experts can provide personalized advice, consider individual needs, and help develop sustainable, health-promoting eating habits. In conclusion, while diets may promise immediate results, their lack of sustainability, exclusionary practices, and potential risks make them a questionable choice for long-term health and well-being. Embracing a balanced, individualized approach to nutrition, supported by professional guidance, can pave the way for lasting success.

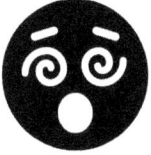

What is the best diet?

The truth is that no diet works for everyone. Did you know that in early Christianity, being fat was considered a sin?

Organic vs. Non-Organic: What You Need to Know to Make Informed Choices

Organic Foods: The U.S. Department of Agriculture (USDA) defines organic foods as fully grown and processed using natural and biological methods, such as soil quality free or minimal pesticide (a harmful chemical linked to many health issues), organic meat and organic animal products derivates need to feed 100% organic forage and food, no hormones, and no antibiotics exempt when the animal becomes sick. These animals should have access to outdoor areas like their natural environment. Federal regulations guidelines state that processed foods to be labeled as organic have to be free from artificial preservatives, artificial fertilizers, artificial coloring, artificial flavors, genetically modified (GM, also known as GMO=genetically modified organisms) and required to have naturally sourced ingredients with minimal exemptions.

When it comes to choosing what we put on our plates, the decision between organic and non-organic foods is a topic that has sparked much debate. The U.S. Department of Agriculture (USDA) defines organic foods as grown and processed using natural and biological methods; this encompasses factors such as soil quality, pesticide use, and the treatment of animals in organic farming practices.

Pros: Firstly, they provide a wealth of nutrients without the harmful chemicals found in conventionally farmed produce. Choosing a diet rich in fresh, delicious foods tastes better and significantly lowers the risk of various cancers, boosts energy levels, enhances concentration, and reduces mental fog by heightened mental clarity and improved overall mood and mental health. Additionally, this wholesome approach diminishes symptoms of depression (related to harmful additives and chemicals added to food) and lessens the likelihood of antibiotic-resistant organisms. Organic farming practices reduce the reliance on antibiotics used in animals.

Moreover, organic farming supports a more vibrant ecosystem, which is crucial for a balanced and sustainable ecosystem, benefiting humankind and the planet while decreasing water contamination from pesticide-related toxins. This nutritional choice also provides abundant essential nutrients, making it a win-win for you and the environment. Finally, organic farming practices help reduce water contamination by removing harmful pesticides that can leach toxins into the environment.

Beyond health, organic produce boasts a superior taste due to healthier soil and more natural growing methods and is generally richer in essential nutrients. Locally grown food and produce typically are the best options. Farmers markets can be fun, and if it is not fun for you, you can feel better by helping the world reduce greenhouse emissions by buying local products and reducing transportation and handling issues. The best practice is farm-to-table whenever possible.

Many people often assert that changing the food system is an unconquerable task. To them, I respond that as long as individuals refrain from educating themselves and remain unaware of the dangers of additives and questionable substances that infiltrate their daily meals, then yes, change may seem impossible. However, envision this: if people take the initiative to educate themselves, become mindful of their food selections, and prioritize their health, a transformation can occur. The industry will be forced to adapt to the shift in consumer demand towards healthier, harmful, chemical-free, and cleaner food options. This shift will respond to consumer preferences and a necessity for businesses to thrive in a market increasingly attuned to the importance of wholesome, nourishing choices. So, the power to revolutionize the food system lies in our collective minds and hands, driven by informed choices and a commitment to well-being.

Cons: While renowned for their health benefits and eco-friendliness, organic foods come with a few considerations. They tend to be pricier than products made with non-organic ingredients or conventional foods. Additionally, due to the absence of synthetic preservatives, organic products have a shorter shelf life and tend to ripen more quickly than their non-organic counterparts. Despite these factors, many people find organic foods' nutritional and environmental advantages to be well worth the investment.

You possess only one body; money may come and go, but your body remains with you. Therefore, it is imperative to be discerning about the foods you purchase and the substances you permit into your system. Your body is a remarkable mechanism that requires proper nourishment to function optimally. The quality of the fuel you provide directly impacts your energy levels, mental clarity, and overall health. By making health-conscious choices in your food selection, you invest in your present vitality, long-term health, and resilience. This means opting for nutrient-dense, wholesome options that fortify your immune system, support cellular regeneration, and sustain your overall physiological balance.

Ultimately, the choice between organic and non-organic foods is personal, influenced by factors like budget, health considerations, and environmental consciousness. Investing in the quality of your food is an investment in your well-being to prevent many diseases linked to non-organic and GMO options. Supporting local and sustainable agriculture is a positive step towards a healthier you and a healthier planet.

Remember: The decisions you make today can significantly impact your future health. It is essential to make smart choices and prioritize caring for your body above everything else.

"Made with Organic Ingredients" Label: A Closer Look

The "Made with Organic Ingredients" label is a designation used to identify products that contain a significant portion of organic components. While not entirely organic, these products must have a minimum of 70% organic ingredients. This label allows consumers to make informed choices about their purchases.

Minimum Organic Content: For a product to be labeled as "Made with Organic Ingredients," it must contain a minimum of 70% organic ingredients. This guarantees that most of the components used in the product meet organic standards. The remaining 30% of the product may include non-organic substances containing chemical additives. However, the use of genetic engineering practices is prohibited in this category.

Cost-Effectiveness: Products labeled "Made with Organic Ingredients" are typically less expensive than fully organic options, making them a more budget-friendly choice for consumers seeking to incorporate organic elements into their diet.

Balancing Affordability and Quality: This labeling option balances affordability and the desire for organic ingredients. It allows consumers to make conscientious choices based on their preferences and budget.

Genetic Engineering Prohibition: Unlike non-organic products, those labeled "Made with Organic Ingredients" cannot contain genetically modified organisms (GMOs); this offers consumers a degree of assurance regarding the source of the ingredients.

Consumer Empowerment: The "Made with Organic Ingredients" label allows consumers to make informed purchasing decisions based on organic content.

The "Made with Organic Ingredients" label offers a valuable middle ground for consumers who are conscious of their dietary choices. While not entirely organic, products bearing this label represent a significant step towards incorporating more organic elements into one's diet. This option is both budget-friendly and allows for informed decision-making, providing consumers with the flexibility to choose products that align with their preferences and values.

Non-Organic Foods: A Detailed Overview

Non-organic foods are produced using conventional farming methods that rely on synthetic chemicals, pesticides, artificial additives, and genetically modified organisms (GMOs). While these practices help ensure a consistent and ample food supply to meet global demands, they come with their own set of advantages and disadvantages.

Pros: Non-organic foods tend to be more cost-effective than their organic counterparts, making them accessible to a wider range of consumers.

Extended Shelf Life: Non-organic foods often have a longer shelf life due to the use of synthetic preservatives. This can reduce food waste and provide greater convenience for consumers.

Potential for Reduced Microbial Growth: Synthetic materials used in non-organic farming may help prevent or reduce the growth of harmful bacteria and molds. This can contribute to food safety.

Nutritional Profile: Some studies suggest that the nutritional content of non-organic foods may be comparable to organic foods. However, it's important to consider the source of these studies and potential biases.

Cons: Harmful and synthetic chemicals used in non-organic farming have been associated with neurotoxic effects, negatively impacting the nervous system.

Endocrine Disruption: Chemical residues in non-organic foods have the potential to disrupt hormonal balance, leading to a range of endocrine-related issues, including issues with the female and male reproductive systems.

Antibiotic Resistance: The use of antibiotics in non-organic farming can contribute to the development of antibiotic-resistant bacteria, posing a significant public health concern.

Increased Cancer Risk: Studies suggest that consumption of certain non-organic foods may be associated with an increased risk of various cancers, including lung, skin, gastrointestinal, breast, prostate, leukemia, and kidney cancers. Clinical studies have revealed a startling finding: certain cancers may manifest up to three generations later because of the genetic mutations induced by harmful chemicals and pesticides.

This indicates the far-reaching impact that our choices today can have on the health of future generations. The implications are profound, emphasizing the critical need for informed decision-making regarding the foods we consume and the agricultural practices we support. By opting for organic produce and products, we take a significant step towards safeguarding not only our own well-being but also that of our descendants. This knowledge empowers us to make choices that resonate across time to a healthier and more resilient legacy for future generations.

Environmental Pollution: Pesticide residues from non-organic farming practices can contribute to environmental pollution, potentially affecting soil, water, and wildlife.

Choosing between organic and non-organic foods involves considering various factors, including budget, health concerns, and environmental considerations. While non-organic foods offer affordability and longer shelf life, they also come with potential health and environmental risks associated with synthetic harmful chemicals and harmful additives. Consumers are encouraged to make informed decisions based on their individual priorities and values.

The Dirty Dozen & Clean Fifteen: A Guide to Pesticides in Produce

The Environmental Working Group (EWG) compiles an annual list of fruits and vegetables known as the "Dirty Dozen" and "Clean Fifteen." These lists are based on data from the U.S. Department of Agriculture (USDA) and Food and Drug Administration (FDA) regarding pesticide residues found on various produce items. This information serves as a guide for consumers who are concerned about their pesticide exposure.

March 2023: The Dirty Dozen

The "Dirty Dozen" includes fruits and vegetables with the highest levels of pesticide residues, even after washing or scrubbing. In 2023, samples from 46,569 pieces of produce were tested, revealing traces of at least 251 different pesticides. Here are the items that ranked highest: strawberries, spinach, kale (collard and mustard greens), peaches, pears, nectarines, apples, grapes, bell and hot peppers, cherries, blueberries, green beans.

March 2023: The Clean Fifteen

The "Clean Fifteen" consists of fruits and vegetables found to have low to negligible traces of pesticides. These items are generally considered safer options, even when conventionally grown. Here is the list for 2023: avocados, sweet corn, pineapple, onions, honeydew melon, asparagus, sweat peas (frozen), papaya, kiwi, cabbage, mushrooms, mangoes, carrots, watermelon, sweet potatoes.

While washing, scrubbing, and peeling fresh produce can reduce pesticide residues, it does not eliminate them. To further minimize exposure, consumers are encouraged to buy organic whenever possible. Additionally, maintaining a diverse diet of fruits and vegetables can help distribute potential pesticide exposure across a range of items. By using the Dirty Dozen and Clean Fifteen as a reference, individuals can make informed choices about which produce items to prioritize.

Optimizing Your Produce Shopping

Exploring various avenues for sourcing fresh and locally produced food can greatly enhance both your diet and your community's well-being.

Farmers markets are vibrant hubs where you can obtain incredibly fresh produce while forging connections with local growers. For those seeking economical options, joining a local food cooperative provides access to organic and locally sourced goods at discounted rates, though do keep in mind the potential for an annual membership fee. Community Supported Agriculture (CSA) programs offer another fantastic opportunity to directly support nearby farms by subscribing to regular deliveries of their bounty, often proving more cost-effective than individual purchases.

Engaging in a community garden, if available, is a gratifying way to cultivate your own produce or partake in collective gardening endeavors; if none exists in your vicinity, consider initiating one! Finally, embracing seasonal buying practices ensures you enjoy the freshest offerings at lower costs. Explore local farmer markets and CSA programs to discover a wealth of seasonal treasures.

Remember, labels like "organic" or "healthy" don't always guarantee that a product is truly organic or beneficial. Always aim for reliable sources such as "Certified Organic," "USDA Certified Organic," and "Certified Organic Non-GMO Project." Consider the Dirty Dozen and Clean Fifteen lists to make informed choices about which produce items to prioritize as organic.

Your health and well-being are worth the extra effort! Accessing fresh and locally sourced produce is beneficial for personal health and for supporting local economies and sustainable agriculture practices.

Finding Farmers Markets: Finding local farmers markets has never been easier. A swift internet search with the query "Farmers Markets near me" can swiftly reveal the closest markets. Additionally, online directories such as LocalHarvest, USDA Farmers Market Directory, and Yelp specialize in cataloging farmer markets, offering a wealth of information, including operating hours and contact details. If your area lacks farmers' markets, take the initiative to start one.

Starting a Farmers Market: Organizing a thriving farmers market involves several key steps. Firstly, engage with your community to assess interest and identify potential vendors, be they local farmers, artisans, or food producers. Next, acquaint yourself with local regulations and permitting requirements, ensuring all necessary permits are obtained from local authorities. Secure an appropriate location, such as a public park or community center, with sufficient space for vendors, visitors, and parking. Diversify vendor selection by reaching out to local growers, artisans, and food producers. Effective promotion through channels like flyers, social media, and local newspapers, as well as creating a dedicated online presence, can significantly broaden the market's reach. Consider adding engaging activities like cooking demonstrations, live music, or educational workshops to enhance the market experience and draw in more visitors. With these steps in place, you'll be well on your way to a successful farmer's market.

Learning from YouTube and Libraries: The journey of starting and managing a farmer's market involves gathering knowledge from diverse sources. YouTube stands out with a treasure of tutorials covering vital aspects like vendor recruitment, market layout, and effective marketing strategies. It's a convenient platform to visually absorb essential information. Additionally, don't underestimate the power of local libraries. These institutions are often stocked with a wealth of resources for community development, event planning, and small-scale entrepreneurship. From informative books and magazines to online materials, libraries offer a well-rounded education on the ins and outs of organizing and managing a successful farmers' market.

Virtual Farmer Groups: Engaging with online farmer communities through forums and social media groups is a fantastic way to tap into a wealth of experience. Platforms like Reddit, Facebook Groups, and specialized agricultural forums provide spaces where you can seek valuable advice, share your experiences, and learn from seasoned individuals. It is important, of course, to always prioritize safety by adhering to group guidelines and avoiding sharing personal information with strangers. Additionally, consider attending webinars and workshops offered by agricultural organizations and institutions. These online events cover various topics relevant to farming, farmer markets, and sustainable agriculture. Participating in such sessions enhances your knowledge base and expands your network within the agricultural community.

By taking these steps, you can enjoy the benefits of fresh, local produce and contribute to building a stronger, more sustainable community. Starting or supporting a farmer's market creates a sense of community, promotes sustainable agriculture, and provides a platform for local businesses to thrive.

Understanding the Impact on Health and Environment GMO vs non-GMO

The topic of GMOs (genetically modified organisms) versus non-GMOs (non-genetically modified organisms) is significant in the food and agriculture industry.

Non-GMO Foods

Natural Cultivation: Non-GMO foods are produced using natural breeding and cultivation methods without genetic modification.

Consumer Preference: Many consumers prefer non-GMO foods due to concerns about potential health risks and the desire for a more "natural" or traditional approach to agriculture.

Organic Certification: Non-GMO foods are often associated with organic farming practices. While organic foods are not necessarily always non-GMO, they do follow similar principles of natural cultivation and avoid genetic modification.

Health Considerations: Advocates for non-GMO foods claim they can be a healthier option, arguing that genetically modified organisms may pose risks such as increased allergenicity, toxicity, and antibiotic resistance.

Environmental Impact: Some proponents argue that non-GMO farming practices can be more environmentally sustainable, as they may use fewer synthetic inputs like pesticides and herbicides.

Genetic Modified Organism (GMO) Foods

Genetic Modification: GMOs are organisms whose genetic material has been altered in a way that does not occur naturally through mating or recombination; this is typically done in a laboratory setting.

Agronomic Benefits: GMOs are often engineered to have specific traits that make them more resistant to pests, diseases, or environmental conditions. For example, some genetically modified crops are designed to withstand herbicides, allowing for more effective weed control.

Food Security and Yield: GMOs are credited with increasing agricultural productivity, allowing for higher yields of crops to meet the demands of a growing global population.

Nutritional Enhancement: Some GMOs are engineered to have enhanced nutritional profiles, which can be particularly important in regions where certain nutrient deficiencies are common.

Controversy and Regulation: The use of GMOs is a highly debated topic. Critics raise concerns about potential unforeseen consequences on the environment and human health, as well as issues of corporate control over food production.

Complexities

Ongoing Research: The long-term effects of GMO consumption on human health and the environment are still being studied, and opinions within the scientific community can vary.

Ethical Considerations: Beyond science, using GMOs also raises ethical questions about owning genetic material, patenting life forms, and equitable access to advanced agricultural technologies.

Coexistence: GMO and non-GMO crops are a practical challenge for farmers, as genetic material can spread through natural processes like pollination. The debate over GMOs versus non-GMOs is multifaceted and involves considerations of food safety, environmental impact, agricultural practices, and ethical concerns. Consumers must stay informed about these issues and make choices that align with their values and beliefs about food production.

Water: In the hydration chapter, you determined the importance of water. Why is water important to you?

_____

_____

_____

_____

Food Groups for Optimal Physiological Performance

Proteins: They are often called building blocks of life because they help create, repair, and replace body organs and cells for growth and optimal functioning. Proteins are not typically used for energy, but when not enough calories are ingested, proteins are broken down into ketones (the body uses its share of savings to sustain life, an approach used on Keto and low-carb diets). A diet high in protein and low in fiber can cause constipation. On the other hand, inadequate protein intake can result in muscle loss, weakening the body's ability to maintain and repair tissues; this can lead to impaired healing and increased susceptibility to infections. Additionally, the immune system may be compromised due to a lack of antibodies primarily composed of proteins. The risk of nutrient deficiency also rises, as protein-rich foods often contain essential vitamins and minerals. Fatigue, weakness, and edema may occur due to the body's struggle to produce sufficient energy and maintain fluid balance. Hair, skin, and nail health can also be negatively impacted, as proteins are essential for their growth and strength. Furthermore, hormonal imbalance, cognitive function impairment, and reduced enzyme activity are potential consequences of insufficient protein intake. Therefore, it is crucial to consider and plan diets involving protein carefully.

Vitamins: Indispensable organic compounds are crucial for various biochemical processes within the human body. They play a pivotal role in supporting growth and development. Essential for nutrient absorption, they enable the body to extract vital elements from our food. B vitamins, including B6, B12, and folic acid, regulate metabolism, converting food into energy and overseeing various metabolic functions. Additionally, vitamins act as antioxidants, safeguarding cells from the harm caused by free radicals, thereby maintaining healthy cellular function and averting oxidative stress. They also fortify the immune system with vitamins C, D, and zinc enhancing the body's defense against infections and illnesses. Furthermore, vitamins are instrumental in tissue repair and wound healing.

For instance, vitamin K is indispensable in blood clotting, expediting wound recovery. Vital for vision, vitamin A aids in the production of retinal pigments, ensuring optimal eye health. Moreover, vitamins D and K are pivotal in fortifying bones, aiding calcium absorption, and ensuring bone density and strength. B vitamins, particularly B6, B9 (folate), and B12, are imperative for neurological function, influencing neurotransmitter synthesis and sustaining a healthy brain. They are also integral to producing red blood cells, preventing anemia, and facilitating proper oxygen transport.

Specific vitamins, such as D, contribute to hormone regulation, impacting the body's production and balance of hormones. A balanced, diverse diet replete with fruits, vegetables, whole grains, lean proteins, and healthy fats is paramount in supplying the body with these vital nutrients. However, supplementation may be advised for individuals with specific dietary needs or medical conditions, always under the guidance of a healthcare professional.

Minerals: Essential nutrients are crucial for various physiological functions, from bone formation and blood clotting to nerve signaling and muscle function. Calcium, for instance, is vital for strong bones and teeth while facilitating proper muscle contraction and blood clotting. Iron is indispensable to produce hemoglobin, the protein in red blood cells that transports oxygen throughout the body. Magnesium supports hundreds of enzymatic reactions, aiding muscles, and nerve function, regulating blood pressure, and maintaining strong bones. Potassium helps regulate blood pressure, balance fluids, and support proper muscle and nerve function.

Zinc is necessary for immune function, wound healing, and DNA synthesis. Copper, on the other hand, is crucial for the formation of connective tissues, as well as for energy production and antioxidant defense. Selenium is an antioxidant, protecting cells from damage and supporting a healthy immune system.

Minerals like sodium, chloride, and potassium are critical in maintaining proper fluid balance and electrolyte levels. A deficiency or excess of these minerals can lead to various health problems, emphasizing the importance of a balanced and varied diet. Fruits, vegetables, whole grains, nuts, seeds, lean proteins, and dairy products are all rich sources of essential minerals. Ensuring an adequate intake of these vital nutrients is essential for preventing deficiencies that can lead to various health issues.

Earth's diverse geological formations host a myriad of minerals, and while there are over 5,000 minerals on Earth, the human body requires a subset of these for its physiological functions. Elements like calcium, potassium, sodium, magnesium, and phosphorus in the Earth's crust and the human body play vital roles in health. Essential trace minerals such as zinc, copper, selenium, and iron, present in Earth's geological makeup, are crucial for enzymatic reactions and cellular function. The interconnectedness extends to nutrient absorption, where plants draw minerals from the soil, and humans, in turn, obtain these minerals by consuming plants. Plants and animals, including humans, obtain essential minerals from the soil and water. Plants absorb minerals from the Earth through their roots. When humans consume these plants, they acquire the minerals for their physiological needs, influenced by regional geological characteristics, diversifying the mineral intake. This evolutionary adaptation emphasizes how humans, as part of the divine design, have developed dietary practices shaped by Earth's mineral offerings, showcasing the profound relationship between the two.

Decoding Carbohydrates

Carbohydrates, a crucial component of our dietary regimen, come in various forms, each wielding distinct effects on our metabolic health. Understanding the interplay between carbohydrates and fats is pivotal in making informed dietary decisions. Know that your brain's preferred energy source is carbohydrates. Your neurons (brain cells) require twice as much energy as the rest of the body cells since the brain cannot store glucose; it depends on what you eat daily. Avoid and or limit foods with high glycemic index (artificial sweeteners, highly processed foods, fast foods, white bread, sugary drinks, white rice, and potatoes, to name a few) that will cause a rapid spike in blood sugar levels, with the result of making you have an energy crash, causing you to be forgetful, fatigued, and foggy.

The Complex Mystery: Complex carbohydrates from whole grains, fruits, and vegetables furnish sustained energy without the rapid spikes in blood sugar levels often associated with refined counterparts.

Carbs: Good vs Bad guys. Starch: Imagine your body as a high-performance car, always needing fuel to run smoothly. Usually, it relies on a type of fuel called glucose, which comes from the food you eat. However, what if there is a shortage of glucose, like at night when you are sleeping or on a special diet? Well, that is when your body has a clever backup plan. It starts using a different kind of fuel called ketones. These ketones are like special energy packs made from your fat! They are created in a special workshop inside you called the liver, where fats are transformed into these super-useful ketone units.

When you are not eating, your insulin levels (the glucose traffic controllers) take a break, but other hormones like glucagon and epinephrine step up to keep things balanced. They send out a message to release fat from storage so it can be turned into ketones. These ketones then travel in your blood, delivering energy to all body parts, like muscles, to keep everything running smoothly. So, think of ketones as your body's secret stash of energy, always there to keep you going, even when the usual fuel supply is running low. It is like having a reserve tank in your car, ensuring you never run out of fuel on your life's journey.

Storytime: The Wise Grain and the Weary Mind

Once upon a time, in a busy village, a wise old grain named Quinoa lived. Quinoa was cherished for its knowledge and revered for its ability to provide energy to those who consumed it.

One sunny day, as Quinoa basked in the golden fields, it noticed a weary traveler named Liam approaching. Liam's face was etched with fatigue, and their steps were heavy with exhaustion. Concerned, Quinoa asked, "Dear traveler, why do you carry the world's weight on your shoulders?"

With a sigh, Liam replied, "I seek clarity of mind and strength to carry on. However, alas, I find myself weary and drained."

Quinoa nodded knowingly and spoke, "Fear not, for I hold the secret to invigorating both body and mind. You see, within me lies the power of carbohydrates, the brain's preferred fuel. When consumed, I break down into glucose, providing immediate energy for your weary mind without needing conversion."

Eager to learn, Liam listened as Quinoa continued, "You must understand, dear traveler, that the brain is a mighty energy consumer, demanding a constant supply to function at its best. Deprivation can lead to weariness, difficulty concentrating, and even memory woes."

Eyes widening in realization, Liam asked, "Is there more to your wisdom, dear Quinoa?"

"Indeed," replied Quinoa, "for I hold the key to another treasure - serotonin, the precursor of good mood. It is a neurotransmitter that can lift the spirits and bring light to even the darkest days."

However, Quinoa's expression grew solemn as it cautioned, "Yet heed this warning, dear traveler. Not all grains are equal. Beware the temptations of processed sugars and refined grains, which lead to fleeting highs and crushing lows. Seek instead the embrace of complex carbohydrates -

bountiful fruits, vibrant vegetables, and steadfast whole grains. They offer a sustained wellspring of energy, like a river that flows steadily."

With understanding, Liam thanked Quinoa for its invaluable lessons. From that day forward, armed with the wisdom of the wise grain, Liam's nourishment and mindful consumption journey flourished, his mind grew sharper, and his spirit soared high, for they had learned the secret of feeding both body and soul.

And so, the tale of Quinoa and the Weary Mind was passed down through the ages, a reminder that our choices in nourishing our bodies echo in the clarity of our thoughts and the radiance of our hearts. The end!

Fats

Often misunderstood, they are crucial for the human body's overall health and proper functioning. They serve as a concentrated energy source, providing twice as many calories per gram as carbohydrates and proteins. This energy reserve proves essential for various bodily functions, including physical activity and metabolic processes. Additionally, fats are crucial in absorbing fat-soluble vitamins (A, D, E, and K), which are necessary for blood clotting, immune function, and bone health. Fats also serve as vital components of cell membranes, aiding in cell structure and function. Omega-3 and omega-6 fatty acids, considered essential fats, cannot be produced by the body and must be obtained through diet. These fatty acids play a key role in brain development, immune function, and reducing inflammation.

Furthermore, fats contribute to producing hormones, including those that regulate metabolism, support growth, and maintain reproductive health. Healthy fats, such as those found in avocados, nuts, seeds, and fatty fish, provide various benefits, from reducing inflammation to supporting heart health and striking a balance between different types of fats while limiting trans and saturated fats.

Omega-3 Fatty acids are a specialized type of lipid present in nearly every cell of our body. They serve as an energy source for our cells, lower the likelihood of blood clot formation, and diminish inflammation, among numerous other functions. Dietary fat constitutes a vital element of human nutrition, an essential macronutrient for all of us. Unlike other fats, omega-3s are crucial in our diet because our bodies cannot produce them independently. Ensuring a diverse intake of various fat types, including omega-3s, can mitigate the risk of deficiency. These fatty acids can be sourced from plants and animals and are also available in supplement form. Fish, seafood, nuts, and plant-based oils are the richest dietary sources. Extensive research on omega-3s has demonstrated their positive impacts on a range of health aspects, spanning from cognitive function to cardiovascular well-being, and they also play a role in various preventive health measures.

Omega-6: Fatty acids play vital roles in bodily functions like cell growth and brain function, but excess can lead to inflammation. Maintaining balance with omega-3 fatty acids is crucial. Both compete for enzymes involved in producing eicosanoids (signaling molecules tied to inflammation). When omega-6 outweighs omega-3, it may lead to chronic inflammation and associated health issues. Both can be balanced through whole foods like fatty fish, nuts, seeds, and greens while minimizing processed foods with omega-6-rich oils. Most omega-6 fatty acids constitute 5% to 10% of daily caloric intake. However, exceeding this range, especially during pregnancy and breastfeeding, may lead to complications. Children above one year typically include omega-6 in their diets, but caution is advised regarding medicinal supplements. Those with COPD should avoid omega-6 supplements, as they can worsen breathing difficulties. Similarly, individuals with high triglycerides or diabetes should be cautious, as omega-6 can elevate triglyceride levels and blood pressure. Overall, prudent consumption of omega-6 is advised for specific health conditions.

Saturated Fats: Type of dietary fat that is typically solid at room temperature. They are found in various animal products like meat, butter, cheese, and dairy products, as well as in some plant oils like coconut oil and palm oil. While for many years, saturated fats were demonized as contributors to heart disease, recent research has provided a more nuanced understanding.

Consuming high amounts of saturated fats, mainly processed and fried foods, can raise LDL cholesterol (often called "bad" cholesterol) levels in the blood, a risk factor for heart disease. However, it is important to note that not all saturated fats are created equal. For instance, high in saturated fats, coconut oil also contains medium-chain triglycerides (MCTs) that may have potential health benefits.

Regarding dietary recommendations, it is advised to consume saturated fats in moderation; this means opting for lean cuts of meat, incorporating more sources of unsaturated fats (like avocados, nuts, and olive oil) into the diet, and being mindful of portion sizes.

Monounsaturated fats are a type of healthy dietary fat that is liquid at room temperature but may solidify when refrigerated. They are considered one of the healthier types of fats and are known for their heart-protective benefits.

Foods rich in monounsaturated fats include:

Olive Oil is the most well-known source of monounsaturated fats. It is a Mediterranean cuisine staple for cooking and dressing.

Avocado: Avocados are not only delicious but are also a great source of monounsaturated fats. They can be added to salads and sandwiches or enjoyed independently.

Nuts: Almonds, cashews, pecans, and macadamia nuts are high in monounsaturated fats. They make for a convenient and nutritious snack.

Seeds: Pumpkin seeds and sesame seeds are good sources of these healthy fats. They can be sprinkled on salads and yogurt or incorporated into various dishes.

Olives are rich in monounsaturated fats and contain various other beneficial nutrients. They are used in salads, spreads, and pizza and pasta toppings.

Peanut Butter: Natural peanut butter (without added sugars or hydrogenated oils) is a tasty way to get monounsaturated fats.

Consuming monounsaturated fats in place of saturated and trans fats can have positive effects on heart health. They have been associated with lowering LDL cholesterol levels and reducing the risk of heart disease. Including various foods can contribute to a balanced and heart-healthy eating pattern. However, while they are healthy, they are also calorie-dense, so moderation is key.

Triglyceride Dilemma: Elevated triglyceride levels, often associated with low-fat diets and rich in carbohydrates, have been linked to increased risks of cardiovascular diseases; this underscores the necessity for a balanced approach where fats and carbohydrates are stable.

Balanced Nutrition Balance emerges as a guiding principle in pursuing health and well-being. Opting for a judicious combination of macronutrients – healthy fats, complex carbohydrates, and lean proteins – promotes metabolic harmony.

Fats: Quality over Quantity

While limiting overall fat intake, the emphasis should be on incorporating wholesome, unsaturated fats such as those found in avocados, nuts, and olive oil. This prudent approach ensures that essential fatty acids are not sacrificed in the quest for a low-fat diet.

Storytime: Friends and Foes in Your Food Adventure

Once upon a time, in the land of Nutritionville, there were special characters called Fats. They were like little helpers in our bodies, giving us energy and keeping our brains smart. Nevertheless, not all fats were the same. Some were like superheroes, and others were tricky.

Meet the Good Fats first! Monounsaturated Fats, found in avocados, nuts, and olive oil, are like the guardians of our hearts. They are heart-friendly and ensure that our hearts stay strong and healthy.

Polyunsaturated Fats were the brainy buddies. They lived in fish, walnuts, and seeds. These fats help our brains think clearly and make our skin glow.

Omega-3 Fatty Acids were the ocean heroes. They lived in fish like salmon and in flaxseeds. Omega-3s were like magic for our hearts and made sure they beat happily.

But then, there were the Tricky Fats!

Saturated Fats are a bit like party crashers. They live in red meat and butter. Too many of them can make our hearts sad and lead to problems.

Trans Fats were sneaky spies. They hid in some processed foods and confused our bodies. They were very tricky and could cause trouble for our hearts.

So, the wise people of Nutritionville learned to choose their foods wisely. They invited the Good Fats to their meals and politely asked the Tricky Fats to stay away. This way, they stayed strong, smart, and healthy!

And they all lived happily ever after, making delicious and nutritious daily choices. The end!

Dietary Fiber

Often referred to as bulk. It is a type of carbohydrate that the body cannot digest, passing through the digestive system mostly intact. There are two main types of dietary fiber: soluble and insoluble. Soluble fiber dissolves in water and forms a gel-like substance, which can help lower cholesterol levels and regulate blood sugar. Insoluble fiber, on the other hand, adds bulk to the stool and aids in regular bowel movements. Both types contribute to maintaining good digestive health.

Additionally, a high-fiber diet can promote a feeling of fullness, making it beneficial for weight management. Fiber-rich foods include fruits, vegetables, whole grains, legumes, and nuts. Integrating a variety of fiber sources into your diet can positively impact your overall health. Remember to increase your fiber intake gradually and stay well-hydrated to support a healthy digestive system.

Sugar - An Enemy or A Friend?

Before the widespread cultivation of sugarcane, honey reigned as the primary natural sweetener. This golden nectar was desired for its natural sweetness and versatility for millennia. Ancient civilizations from Egypt to Greece held honey in high regard, utilizing it not only as a sweetener but also as a vital ingredient in various culinary and medicinal preparations. Its production involved the remarkable work of honeybees, which transformed nectar from flowering plants into this cherished substance through a complex process of regurgitation and evaporation. The rich history of honey reflects humanity's deep-seated appreciation for the gifts of nature.

Sugar was a rare and luxurious indulgence in its early days, primarily accessible to the elite and affluent. Its value was so esteemed that it was often considered a form of medicine. This precious commodity was initially harvested from sugarcane, a tall grass native to New Guinea, and its cultivation quickly spread to regions like India, where its production dates to the 4th century BC. As the demand for sugar surged, so did its significance in global trade, shaping economies and influencing cultural exchanges. By the 15th century, with Portuguese explorers' exploration of the Atlantic islands, sugar found a new heaven for cultivation, forever altering its accessibility and setting the stage for a new chapter in its history.

Unfortunately, this period also saw the reprehensible practice of African slavery in sugar-producing colonies. Christopher Columbus brought sugarcane to the Caribbean in the late 15th century, establishing a flourishing industry powered by forced labor. This era marked the inception of the Atlantic triangular trade, profoundly reshaping history. Following the abolition of slavery, indentured laborers, primarily from India, took their place, leading to significant demographic shifts. Sugar became a vital energy source for laborers during the Industrial Revolution, and later, mechanization in the 1900s led to a surplus of sugar, contributing to its widespread incorporation into processed foods today. The journey of sugar exemplifies its enduring demand, steering societal transformations and leaving an indelible imprint on our world.

It is essential to understand that excessive sugar intake can be perilous for health, often leading to various illnesses, one of the most prevalent being type 2 diabetes. This chronic condition, over time, puts immense strain on the body's organs, eventually leading them to become overworked and fatigued, which can result in organ failure. Throughout my career, I have witnessed not just isolated cases of diabetes but rather diabetic patients struggling with three or more concurrent health issues.

Given the efforts required by the brain, kidneys, and heart to combat insulin resistance, many people with diabetes eventually face conditions like neuropathy, kidney dysfunction, heart complications, limb amputations, heart disease, eye diseases, cancer, and many other diseases secondary to diabetes.

It is worth noting that diabetes significantly hampers the body's healing process after surgeries or injuries. Interestingly, it is a two-way street; sometimes, diabetes arises as a secondary consequence of an underlying condition, medications, or poor lifestyle choices, or vice versa. The vivid memories of these experiences are engraved into my mind like a three-dimensional model, serving as a powerful reminder of the importance of managing sugar intake. However, its effects on the body are far from sweet. Sugar is a pervasive presence in our diets, permeating all processed foods. The prevalence of high fructose corn syrup, 1.5 times sweeter than table sugar, further exacerbates the issue.

When we consume sugar, the small intestine converts it into Very low-density lipoproteins (VLDL), which then the muscles and fat cells convert into Low-Density Lipoproteins or LDL for short ("bad cholesterol") to prevent it from entering the liver. Instead, it enters the bloodstream as LDL cholesterol, a mechanism designed to shield the liver. However, excessive sugar intake overwhelms the small intestine's capacity, flooding the liver; this triggers a cascade of problems, from oxidative stress to insulin resistance and mitochondrial dysfunction. The overburdened liver prompts the pancreas to work harder to compensate.

This relentless cycle dramatically heightens the risk of debilitating conditions such as type 2 diabetes, cardiovascular disease, dyslipidemia, dementia, cancer, polycystic ovarian disease, hypertension, and fatty liver disease, which, unfortunately, lack a definitive cure. However, a powerful antidote lies in adopting a non-negotiable commitment to a healthier lifestyle. By making mindful choices about your diet, you hold the key to preventing these chronic illnesses and unlocking a healthier future.

Are you ready for an unappetizing real story?

No worries, I try to be as professional as possible and not give you too many details that will freak you out. Pinky promises that I will keep the story PG-13. The most atypical stories are from non-compliant patients who do not follow their treatment plan for one reason or another. And then, of course, their condition deteriorates. So, here I was, caring for this young man in his early 20s. He had a couple of autoimmune diseases and secondary type 2 diabetes. He was non-compliant and paraplegic (paralysis from the waist down). He developed multiple stage four wounds (meaning you could see the bones, and they were full of pus and dead cells, with a strong foul odor that wafted to the entrance door). He underwent multiple surgeries to repair the wounds, which worked for many of them, but six of them remained and got constantly infected, causing him to be in the hospital for months multiple times. His buttocks wound was so big that it covered both cheeks. Man, those wounds were like a labyrinth! I had to pack them, and I could see half of my right hand disappear inside them (I have taken care of patients where my whole hand to my wrist disappeared in there), so that was nothing to me. This patient had already endured so much pain and suffering—from a traumatic childhood to a chronically ill youth to a deadly adulthood. He was recommended to have below-the-knee amputations on both legs. We tried everything to help those wounds heal.

172

When I took over his case, I was warned about how rude, disrespectful, non-compliant, and foul-mouthed he was and how he had tried to take his life multiple times. This patient knew diabetes top to bottom and knew a lot more about it than many clinicians he encountered. So, from day one, he started quizzing me and trying to be disrespectful, cursing left and right. However, I was a knowledgeable nurse, and most of the time, he got defensive when I was educating him about his disease and the lifestyle choices he had to make to improve his condition. He was not having it because he knew what he had to do very well.

Moreover, his meal options were limited since he was unemployed and on food stamps. He tried to find every excuse possible, but I always had my punch line and outsmarted him with love, kindness, and understanding. Eventually, his wounds started to get better to the point where he did not need the wound VAC (vacuum-assisted wound closure, which works for some patients and others it does not) on his buttocks wound. He became a candidate for surgery, but the wounds on his legs got severely infected, resulting in one of his heels developing necrotizing fasciitis (flesh-eating disease). The disease was so bad that all the heel skin was missing, but he continued to refuse to go to the hospital. Finally, I could reason with him and get his hinny to the hospital. After that, I am unsure what happened to him, but I highly doubt he is among the living. This patient's story is a reminder of the importance of making healthier choices to prevent chronic illnesses.

Necrotizing fasciitis is a rare but deadly bacterial infection that spreads quickly under the skin. It is caused by bacteria that enter the body through a break in the skin, such as a cut, wound, scrape, or burn. The bacteria can also enter the body through surgery or an infection. The initial signs often include redness, swelling, and a noticeable warmth at the site of the infection, indicating the body's immediate response to the invading pathogens. As the condition progresses, severe pain becomes apparent, reflecting the severity of the tissue damage. In advanced stages, one may observe the formation of blisters or even black sores, indicating significant tissue necrosis (tissue death). Systemic symptoms like fever and chills also arise, signaling the body's systemic response to the infection. Necrotizing fasciitis is a medical emergency and requires prompt treatment.

Calories-The Good, Bad, and Ugly

The term "Calorie" was first introduced in 1819 by Nicolas Clément, a French chemistry professor. Clément used the term calorie to explain how steam engines convert heat into work. Fast-forward to 1873-1907, another chemistry professor named Wilbur O. Atwater introduced Americans to a new unit of energy in food (aka Calorie, but calorie and Calorie are not the same thing but do not worry, I will not talk about that). Atwater used a bomb calorimeter to come up with the calories in foods. To this day, some food calories may vary from his original measurements, but the idea behind it is still relatively the same in terms of giving us an idea of how to measure the energy in the foods we ingest.

Now, are you ready for this? Calorie counting should not be your sole focus. It is often not worth the headache and is not even sustainable. I like to pay attention to calories to determine if a typical food or product is good for me. However, I pay even more attention to the ingredient list to decide. This way, I can see beyond deceiving products and often misleading marketing practices.

When traveling to countries around the world, I have encountered various units of energy measurement, such as Kilocalories (Kcal), Calorie (with an uppercase 'C'), calorie (with a lowercase' c'), joules (J), and Kilojoules (Kj). It is worth noting that one calorie is equivalent to 4 joules. Understanding these units can be beneficial, particularly when managing your caloric intake and expenditure for weight management. However, it is important to consider whether your goal is overall weight loss or specifically reducing body fat percentage, as they can have different implications, including potential plateaus in progress.

On the other hand, it is interesting to reflect on the origins of these units since they were devised in physics and chemistry to quantify the energy usage of machines. While the human body operates similarly, a certain level of abstraction is involved.

In a somewhat ironic twist, in 1948, the scientific community declared both 'Calorie' and 'calorie' outdated. The reason? They simply needed to be more precise. This led to a shift towards adopting the joule as the standard energy measurement unit. Many countries made this transition, recognizing the clarity it offered.

However, it is worth noting that the United States, among a few others, still predominantly employs the term 'Calorie' in dietary contexts. In contrast, numerous countries have seamlessly integrated kilocalories (kcal) and joules into their product packages. This diverse landscape of energy measurement units indicates the dynamic nature of scientific language and its adaptation across cultures.

Why Should Fruits and Vegetables Be Your Best Friends?

Fresh, ideally organic, fruits and vegetables should be cherished as your closest allies due to their incredible nutritional benefits. In today's fast-paced world, our focus on food has shifted towards its appearance, flavor, and presentation. We often turn to food for solace, allowing it to comfort us rather than truly nourish us. Emotions like happiness, sadness, boredom, and excitement can trigger our eating habits. Food plays multiple roles in our lives. It is a source of celebration and comfort, and sometimes, we treat ourselves just for the sake of it. In this process, many of us have lost sight of the true purpose of food. Instead of appreciating its nutritional value, we may find ourselves in an inner dialogue critiquing its taste or palatability.

Nevertheless, a simple shift in mindset can make all the difference. Acknowledge that each food serves a purpose in nourishing your body. Understand that it contributes to the healthy, vibrant person you are becoming. Your cells thrive on the nutrients it provides. Sometimes, it is true that a particular food may not be your favorite in terms of taste. However, reminding yourself of its immense nutritional value can transform your relationship with it.

7 Strategies to Optimize Your Health & Prevent Chronic Illnesses.

Food is meant to be a source of nourishment, not a trigger for illness. Due to its remarkable intelligence, the human body reacts rapidly upon encountering foreign or harmful substances; this may be why some people experience a decline in health, moving from mild discomfort to more severe issues, especially when the condition becomes chronic with no clear solution.

It is imperative to treat your body like a cherished home, nurturing it with the right foods and the care it deserves. By embracing fresh, wholesome fruits and vegetables, you are enriching your body and fortifying your health in the long run.

Storytime: The Keto Journey-A Tale of Mindful Choices

Once upon a time, in the bustling town of Wellsville, there lived a young woman named Emma. Emma was vibrant and energetic, always eager to explore new horizons. A wave of curiosity washed over her when she heard about the keto diet. She was enticed by the promise of renewed vitality and decided to try it.

As she explored her keto adventure, Emma learned about the potential challenges ahead. She discovered that the initial stages could bring about what was known as the "keto flu." Emma was not discouraged, for she understood that her body was adapting to a new way of fueling itself. With patience and determination, she pushed through, knowing that the discomfort was temporary.

Emma was also mindful of the potential risks associated with the keto diet. If not approached with care, it could lead to low blood pressure, kidney stones, and nutrient deficiencies. Her heart swelled with gratitude for her body, and she resolved to treat it with kindness and respect.

As she continued her keto journey, Emma met a wise old herbalist named Clara. Clara had a wealth of knowledge about holistic health and nutrition. Emma shared her experiences and concerns with Clara, who listened attentively. Clara imparted invaluable advice about staying attuned to her body's signals and seeking balance.

With Clara's guidance, Emma made informed choices about her keto diet. She focused on nutrient-dense foods, ensuring she met her body's needs for vitamins and minerals. She also recognized the importance of regular check-ins with her healthcare provider to monitor her overall health.

Emma's journey had challenges, but she navigated them gracefully and wisely. Like any other dietary approach, she understood that the keto diet was not a one-size-fits-all solution. It required thoughtful consideration and respect for her body's unique needs.

In the end, Emma's story inspired those in Wellsville and beyond. Her mindful approach to the keto diet showed that one could embark on a journey towards better health with knowledge, self-awareness, and guidance. And so, the tale of Emma and her keto adventure became a cherished story, passed down through generations, reminding all who heard it of the power of mindful choices in the pursuit of well-being. The end!

Decoding Labels- The World of Natural Flavors

One ingredient often overlooked is flavor. Artificial flavors, while tempting, can carry hidden risks. They have been associated with hypertension, diabetes, and digestive discomfort. It is a clear call to action - opt for products without these potentially harmful additives.

However, as you become a more discerning consumer, be wary of the term "natural flavors" on labels. Manufacturers may use this term to evoke an image of wholesome ingredients, but the reality can be quite different. Behind the scenes, these so-called "natural flavors." This category encompasses a multitude of laboratory-created compounds, numbering up to 100 or more.

To ensure you make the healthiest choice, seek products that go the extra mile. Look for labels that proudly display "organic" and "non-GMO" certifications. These indicators signal a commitment to quality, transparency, and a genuine concern for your health.

Remember that your choices mark your journey towards better health. By reading into ingredient lists and understanding the nuances of labels, you empower yourself to select supplements that align with your vision of optimal health. Your body will thank you for it.

Understanding Common Ingredients in Everyday Products

Mercury: A Global Health Hazard: Recognized by the World Health Organization as a significant health threat, mercury should have no place in your supplements. Overexposure to mercury can lead to cellular damage and DNA harm. Choosing mercury-free options is a wise step towards a healthier future.

Titanium Dioxide: Found in cosmetics and paint, titanium dioxide is a filler that offers no nutritional value. Its consumption, even in small amounts, can lead to allergies and organ toxicity. The inhalation of titanium dioxide powder can even pose a risk of cancer. opt for supplements without this unnecessary additive.

Magnesium Silicate (Talc): Just as cosmetics are not meant for consumption, neither is talc. It shares a composition with asbestos, making it unsuitable for ingestion. Long-term exposure can lead to stomach issues and lung diseases. Choose supplements free from magnesium silicate.

Artificial Coloring: While artificial colors enhance visual appeal, they come at a price. Linked to hyperactivity in children and a range of health issues, these additives are best avoided. Look for supplements without artificial coloring to prioritize your well-being.

Lead: Surprisingly, lead can find its way into supplements, often used as a colorant, raising concerns, especially for expectant mothers and young children. Lead exposure during pregnancy can affect a child's cognitive and neurobehavioral development. Always check labels and choose products with safe lead levels. Please note that deceitful manufacturers may use lead other names to mask their use; the same holds true for many other ingredients. Set aside some time to get familiar with the ingredient list of products that you frequently buy.

Hydrogenated Oil: Known to elevate "bad cholesterol," hydrogenated oil poses risks to cardiovascular and nervous system health. Follow dietary guidelines and limit your intake of this unhealthy fat.

Supplementation vs Natural Foods

Dietary supplements can be beneficial when sourced from reputable manufacturers to address specific deficiencies. I integrate some supplements into my regimen, but not daily or frequently. It is essential to consider that many supplements undergo similar chemical engineering processes as regular medications. Opting for organically sourced, liquid-form supplements closer to vegan and non-GMO can lead to higher quality products often subject to more rigorous regulation. It is crucial, especially if you are on prescription medications, to check for potential interactions between your supplements and prescribed drugs.

Additionally, scrutinizing the ingredient list is vital, as some supplements may be contaminated with pesticides, heavy metals, or bacteria, particularly those of inferior manufacturing quality. Every supplement has potential side effects, so informed choices are key to ensuring their safety and effectiveness. With mindful selection, you can support your body's optimal performance and recovery. Choose wisely and let your health flourish.

Choosing Supplements Wisely: Many of us turn to supplements to fill potential nutrient gaps in the quest for a healthier, more vibrant life. However, not all supplements are created equal. Being a discerning consumer and knowing what ingredients to avoid is imperative. Make informed choices with supplements with a short ingredient list, minimal chemical components that are not harmful to your health, and as organic as possible. I will help you to get started.

7 Strategies to Optimize Your Health & Prevent Chronic Illnesses.

Food servings and recommendations: The truth is, as plate sizes have expanded, so have our waistlines. In the 1950s, the standard plate size in the USA was around 8.5 to 9 inches. Today, it is common to find plates ranging from 10.5 to 12 inches. It is a simple psychological trick: the larger the plate, the more we tend to serve ourselves. Even if we feel satisfied with food, many of us succumb to finishing it out of guilt. The solution? Get for a smaller plate, ☺. This subtle shift can help regulate portion sizes and promote healthier eating habits. It is not about deprivation but about mindful choices that support our well-being.

Your Body Mass Index (BMI) and Weight Should No Longer Be the Focus

Body mass index (BMI) is a useful tool for determining whether you are underweight, average, or overweight. However, it is important to remember that BMI does not consider factors like muscle mass, body type, or genetic influences. Interestingly, this scale was created in the 1830s by someone who was not a medical doctor, yet it remains in common use today. Designed initially to find the "average man," it does not encompass the diversity of human bodies.

When we step on a scale, we often fixate on its number without considering that it measures our entire body—organs, muscles, water weight, and even waste (aka poop). For the most accurate weight, weigh yourself first thing in the morning or right before bed, with an empty bladder and after a bowel movement (yes, every bit counts!). And do not be shy wearing your birthday suit (nakedness) to the scale ensures the most accurate measurement.

Rather than becoming fixated on your weight, I recommend paying more attention to your body fat percentage; this is a more reliable indicator of your overall health. With today's technology, you can find electronic scales measuring your body fat percentage. However, it is worth noting that some of these scales can be less accurate, so be sure to read reviews before making a purchase. Look for one with an app to track your progress, as these can be found online or even at your doctor's office, nutritionist's clinic, or aesthetic clinic.

Recommendations

Your body's well-being depends on balanced nutrition. Imbalances lead to malnourishment, causing various health issues. In today's fast-paced society, meal timing often needs to be addressed. Irregular eating habits contribute to digestive problems. Establishing a consistent eating routine supports proper body and mind function. For those constantly on the move, having a nutritious, easy-to-digest snack or smoothie can make a significant difference. Here, you will find it quick, satisfying, and delicious.

During meals, pay attention to chewing habits. Be present and mindful of flavors. Avoid distractions from electronic devices and steer clear of stressful situations while eating. Refrain from late-night snacking. Ideally, allow 2 hours before bedtime for digestion to ensure your body can focus on essential processes during sleep rather than digestion.

Additionally, consider waiting 30-60 minutes after waking up before having your first meal, if possible. While this adjustment may pose initial challenges, the long-term benefits are well worth it. Choose nutritious, organic foods that align with your journey towards a healthier you. Maintain your positivity and optimism, striving for progress each day.

Next, I will provide you with some meal recommendations. If you have any medical conditions or are under the care of healthcare professionals, please consult with them first. Always pay attention to how your body feels; this will ensure you promote healthier eating habits without starving yourself.

When it comes to how you eat, your seating posture matters. It improves digestion and helps the body absorb nutrients more efficiently. Taking a few deep breaths before you start eating can also reduce stress levels. Minimizing distractions is important. As for where you get your meals, the best place is at home. When you prepare your meals, you have control over the quantity and quality of the ingredients. If you are a busy bee like me and always on the go, meal prepping can be a lifesaver. When that is not an option, you can do an internet search for places to eat around you offering meals aligning with your healthy eating journey. You can even look at the menu ahead of time.

A Guide to Understanding and Managing Hunger

0- Hungry: No
1- Hungry: Not so much
2- A little hungry
3- Hungry
4- Very Hungry
5- Hungry: Starving

SPOILER ALERT

Make sure you are not at a 5/5 on the hunger scale. If you are, you are more likely to choose options that might not be the best for your healthy journey. Since we all react differently to stressors, the best approach is planning what to eat right after breakfast; this might seem annoying, but in my culture, this way of thinking reduces the stress and anxiety of figuring out what to eat when starving, short on time, or not even in the mood for food.

Pay close attention to how hungry you feel. You might not make the healthiest choice if you wait until you are famished and ready to devour anything in 3 seconds. Planning can make a big difference in maintaining a balanced and nourishing diet.

Satiation Rating

Fullness Scale

1- Full: No
2- Not Really
3- A little Full
4- Full
5- Very Full
6- Too full (stuffed)

Keep in mind: Chew each bite 5-10 times, depending on the type of food. Reduce stress while eating; eliminate electronic devices if possible. It may take 20 minutes for your stomach to tell your brain that it is full. These signals can get interrupted when we do not pay attention to our meals.

Next, I will offer some meal prep recommendations. If you have any medical conditions or are under the care of healthcare professionals, it is important to consult with them first.

Mastering the Art of Meal Preparation for Health and Flavor

Meal prepping in tight glass containers is one of the best options for preserving freshness. Ideally, freeze food for about 1-2 weeks to prevent "freezer burn" and maintain quality and taste. However, you should always do what works best for you.

It is worth noting that the degradation process slows down when you freeze food but does not stop entirely; this can lead to changes in texture, flavor, and color, resulting in food that may not taste as fresh.

When freezing food, it is advisable to do so in portions you will use to avoid any inconvenience later. I recommend using BPA-free seal-tight or airtight storage containers (as BPA has been linked to various health issues like cancer, high blood pressure, type 2 diabetes, and heart diseases). Glass containers with BPA-free lids are a safer alternative. Sealed plastic-free bags are also an acceptable option.

Freezing specific foods like bread, cake, fruits, and vegetables is a convenient way to extend their shelf life. When freezing bread, separating the loaves is a good practice to prevent them from sticking together; this ensures you can easily retrieve a portion when needed. Similarly, cakes can be frozen to preserve their freshness for special occasions. When it comes to fruits and vegetables, freezing can lock in their nutrients, making them an excellent option for later use in smoothies, soups, and other dishes. Proper storage in sealed containers or plastic-free bags helps maintain their quality and flavor. So, with a little preparation, you can make the most of these foods and reduce waste.

Freezing food is an effective way to prevent illness-causing organisms from growing and potentially making you sick. However, it is important to note that these harmful organisms can replicate quickly when frozen foods are thawed.

Certain foods, such as bread, cookies, and pastries, can be safely thawed at room temperature and stored at room temperature afterward. Allowing them to thaw naturally at room temperature ensures they retain their texture and flavor. However, this method is suitable only for items that can withstand room-temperature storage without compromising their quality or safety. Always be mindful of food safety practices to enjoy these treats without concerns.

Thawing certain foods in the refrigerator is a safe practice to prevent the growth of harmful organisms. This method is suitable for vegetables, fruits, meat (which can also be thawed in cold water away from direct sunlight), milk, prepared food, and rice (preferably for reheating after being frozen). Refrigeration maintains a controlled temperature, ensuring these items thaw gradually and safely. By following these guidelines, you can confidently enjoy these foods, knowing they are both delicious and free from potential health risks.

Minimizing microwave usage and opting for stove reheating can enhance your meals' flavor and nutritional value. While the impact of microwaving on food quality is debated among scientists, it is advisable to exercise caution and limit microwave use. Embracing traditional cooking and stove reheating methods connects us to simpler times and offers a chance to savor meals in their most authentic form. By making this small shift, you may find a greater appreciation for the culinary process and the wholesome, nourishing meals it yields.

When reheating food, ensure it reaches a steaming hot temperature and avoid reheating it more than once. It is worth noting that certain foods are best avoided in the microwave due to potential changes in taste or texture. These include chicken, breast milk, processed meats, leafy greens, hot peppers, potatoes, hard-boiled eggs, rice, beets, and fruits. Consider alternative reheating methods for these items for optimal taste and food safety.

After preparing meals, it is important to refrigerate any leftovers within one hour to prevent the multiplication of harmful organisms. When it comes to leftover rice, ensure you consume it within three days and always reheat it until steaming hot to avoid the risk of food poisoning. Taking these precautions will help maintain the safety and quality of meals.

7 Strategies to Optimize Your Health & Prevent Chronic Illnesses.

21 Days Meal Plan

Week 1:

Day 1

Breakfast: Greek yogurt with mixed berries and granola.
Lunch: Turkey and avocado wrap with whole wheat tortilla.
Dinner: Grilled salmon with roasted vegetables.
Snack: Apple slices with almond butter.

Day 2

Breakfast: Oatmeal with banana and cinnamon.
Lunch: Grilled chicken salad with mixed greens, cherry tomatoes, and balsamic vinaigrette.
Dinner: Baked sweet potato topped with black beans, salsa, and avocado.
Snack: Carrot sticks with hummus.

Day 3

Breakfast: Scrambled eggs with spinach and feta cheese.
Lunch: Quinoa and vegetable stir-fry.
Dinner: Turkey chili with cornbread.
Snack: Greek yogurt with honey and walnuts.

Day 4

Breakfast: Smoothie bowl with mixed berries, banana, and granola.
Lunch: Tuna salad with mixed greens and whole wheat crackers.
Dinner: Grilled chicken with quinoa and steamed broccoli.
Snack: Mixed nuts with dried fruit.

Day 5

Breakfast: Whole wheat toast with avocado and smoked salmon.
Lunch: Grilled Portobello mushroom burger on whole wheat bun.
Dinner: Spaghetti squash with turkey meatballs and marinara sauce.
Snack: Apple slices with peanut butter.

Day 6

Breakfast: Greek yogurt with banana, honey, and chia seeds.
Lunch: Chicken and vegetable kebabs with brown rice.
Dinner: Baked salmon with roasted sweet potatoes and asparagus.
Snack: Cherry tomatoes with mozzarella cheese.

Day 7
Breakfast: Veggie omelet with spinach, tomato, and onion.
Lunch: Turkey and vegetable soup with whole wheat bread.
Dinner: Grilled chicken with roasted cauliflower and carrots.
Snack: Sliced pear with almond butter.

Week 2:

Day 8

Breakfast: Overnight oats with mixed berries and almond milk.
Lunch: Grilled chicken and vegetable wrap with whole wheat tortilla.
Dinner: Baked sweet potato topped with grilled shrimp and steamed broccoli.
Snack: Greek yogurt with mixed nuts.

Day 9

Breakfast: Smoothie with banana, almond milk, and peanut butter.
Lunch: Quinoa and vegetable salad with lemon vinaigrette.
Dinner: Grilled chicken with brown rice and roasted vegetables.
Snack: Apple slices with cinnamon.

Day 10

Breakfast: Whole wheat toast with avocado and hard-boiled egg.
Lunch: Grilled Portobello mushroom salad with mixed greens and balsamic vinaigrette.
Dinner: Spaghetti squash with ground turkey and marinara sauce.
Snack: Carrot sticks with hummus.

Day 11

Breakfast: Greek yogurt with mixed berries and granola.
Lunch: Tuna salad with mixed greens and whole wheat crackers.
Dinner: Grilled salmon with roasted sweet potatoes and asparagus.
Snack: Mixed nuts with dried fruit.

Day 12

Breakfast: Scrambled eggs with spinach and feta cheese.
Lunch: Quinoa and vegetable stir-fry.
Dinner: Turkey chili with cornbread.
Snack: Sliced pear with almond butter.

Day 13

Breakfast: Smoothie bowl with mixed berries, banana, and granola.
Lunch: Chicken and vegetable kebabs with brown rice.

Dinner: Baked salmon with roasted cauliflower and carrots.
Snack: Cherry tomatoes with mozzarella cheese.

Day 14

Breakfast: Whole wheat toast with avocado and smoked salmon.
Lunch: Turkey and avocado wrap with whole wheat tortilla.
Dinner: Grilled chicken with quinoa and steamed broccoli.
Snack: Apple slices with peanut butter.

Week 3

Day 15

Breakfast: Veggie omelet with spinach, tomato, and onion.
Lunch: Grilled Portobello mushroom burger on whole wheat bun.
Dinner: Spaghetti squash with turkey meatballs and marinara sauce.
 Snack: Greek yogurt with honey and walnuts.
Day 16

Breakfast: Overnight oats with mixed berries and almond milk.
Lunch: Grilled chicken and vegetable wrap with whole wheat tortilla.
Dinner: Baked sweet potato topped with black beans, salsa, and avocado.
Snack: Carrot sticks with hummus.

Day 17

Breakfast: Smoothie with banana, almond milk, and peanut butter.
Lunch: Quinoa and vegetable salad with lemon vinaigrette.
Dinner: Grilled chicken with brown rice and roasted vegetables.
Snack: Apple slices with cinnamon.

Day 18

Breakfast: Greek yogurt with mixed berries and granola.
Lunch: Tuna salad with mixed greens and whole wheat crackers.
Dinner: Grilled salmon with roasted vegetables.
Snack: Mixed nuts with dried fruit.

Day 19

Breakfast: Scrambled eggs with spinach and feta cheese.
Lunch: Chicken and vegetable kebabs with brown rice.
Dinner: Turkey chili with cornbread.
Snack: Greek yogurt with mixed nuts.

Day 20

Breakfast: Smoothie bowl with mixed berries, banana, and granola.
Lunch: Grilled Portobello mushroom salad with mixed greens and balsamic vinaigrette.
Dinner: Baked sweet potato topped with grilled shrimp and steamed broccoli.
Snack: Sliced pear with almond butter.

Day 21

Breakfast: Whole wheat toast with avocado and hard-boiled egg.
Lunch: Turkey and vegetable soup with whole wheat bread.
Dinner: Grilled chicken with roasted cauliflower and carrots.
Snack: Cherry tomatoes with mozzarella cheese.

These meals are balanced and nutritious and should help you maintain a healthy diet throughout the 21-day challenge. Please remember that this is only a blueprint; feel free to substitute any ingredient based on your dietary preferences.

Your poop says it all.

Stools with a foul odor, which is also known as stinky poop, could be a sign of a digestive medical condition, or it may be related to your diet. When you consume foods that are unsuitable for your body, the poop emits a bad smell because the body's good bacteria start breaking down most of this waste, triggering chemical reactions in your digestive tract to eliminate these foreign substances.

Did you know that your gut is home to a tiny ecosystem that can produce methane gas? It is a fascinating fact that not many people are aware of!

Some individuals produce more methane gas than others. For those with increased methane gas in their digestive system, bloating, abdominal cramping/pain, and constipation can be problematic. The heightened methane gas production in your digestive tract creates an environment conducive to the growth and replication of harmful bacteria in your gut; this alters your gut microbiota, which may lead to illness and prolonged health issues over time.

Body Taxation (BTT)

As a healthcare worker for nearly two decades, I have witnessed thousands of people suffer the consequences of poor lifestyle choices and self-destructive behaviors. However, I must tell you that the most impactful times in my career have been as a hospice nurse. Taking care of terminally ill patients has taught me the importance of how past and present choices affect the future. One of the most heart-wrenching scenarios is when a patient receives a stage 4 cancer diagnosis, and the available treatments would cause more harm than letting nature take its course. So many times, I have heard lung cancer patients say, "I do not know why I got lung cancer; I quit smoking more than 20 years ago." I have cared for people who tried to correct their behaviors, but unfortunately, it was too late for them because their bodies had already presented them with the final bill.

Your body manages your organs like finances. Let me explain this: Your body keeps an open tab of your healthy and unhealthy transactions, understanding that by making poor lifestyle choices, your body becomes heavily taxed. As years of unhealthy decisions accumulate, your body is already tallying up the cells. The problem arises when there are fewer healthy cells and more damaged cells, or the body cannot produce more healthy cells. Your body warns you of what is transpiring inside you. If you do not pay attention and persist with unhealthy habits, eventually, your body hands you the final bill. Luckily, you're here, improving your health and habits, so your body won't tax you the same way it would if you didn't act to better your life.

Consuming more unhealthy meals causes your magnificent body to overwork, become fatigued, and eventually burn out, leading to many diseases. Eating healthy foods is crucial not only for feeling good but also for preventing chronic illnesses. Do not let deceptive marketing sway you. Do your research and ensure the products you purchase and consume come from reputable providers. Many companies label their products as "healthy," "heart-healthy," or "beneficial for this or that," but are they true? Marketing tactics target what is trending. For example, most companies observe that people are becoming more health-conscious and changing their eating habits. They will then create or modify current products with a marketing campaign to entice people to buy. They will employ various psychological tactics. We must be resilient to these marketing strategies and build our immunity against them.

Choices and the Dark Side of Marketing (CDM)

I vividly recall the time before embarking on my health journey. My fluid intake consisted solely of coffee and soda for an extended period. The taste of water was unappealing to me. Each time a commercial for sodas or coffee came on, my brain lit up with anticipation for what I craved and desired.

Even when I tried to adopt a healthier lifestyle, these commercials continued to sway my choices. It was not until I put my foot down and committed myself to prioritizing my well-being that I broke free from their influence.

Marketing serves a positive purpose in informing consumers about various products. However, there is a dark side to marketing. Many companies are solely concerned with their profits and could not care less about consumer health. If these products continue to generate revenue, companies will pour resources into advertising and employ psychological tactics to entice you to buy. In many situations, companies incorporate chemicals designed to induce food cravings, with sugar being one of the most prominent culprits.

Certain chemicals in food products have become a common practice among manufacturers. Manufacturers collaborate with physicists, chemists, and neuroscientists to engineer their products in a way that triggers irresistible cravings in consumers. These cravings are carefully designed to compel you to reach for that second cookie, brownie, or piece of chocolate - whatever your weakness may be. The science behind this manipulation is complex, but the result is a product that is difficult to resist.

What strategies can you employ to shield yourself from the influence of unethical advertisements?

Be aware of the persuasive tactics used in advertisements. Recognize when they are trying to appeal to your emotions or create a sense of urgency.

Create a Shopping List: Before going shopping, make a list of what you need. Stick to it and avoid impulsive purchases prompted by commercials or advertisements on social media.

Limit Screen Time: Limit TV and online streaming to reduce exposure to commercials. Opt for ad-free platforms or use ad blockers.

Educate Yourself: Before purchasing any item, research products independently, read reviews, check ingredient labels, and consider alternatives.

Set Clear Goals: Clarify your health and lifestyle goals to resist temptation.

Practice Delayed Gratification: If you see something advertised, give yourself time to think it over. Avoid making impulsive decisions.

Understand Emotional Triggers: When watching commercials, be aware of emotional manipulation and evaluate if the product is genuinely beneficial.

Seek Recommendations: When making important decisions, seek advice from trustworthy sources like friends and family rather than relying solely on marketing claims.

Prioritize Needs over Wants: Distinguish between needs and wants. Prioritize genuine needs over desires.

Practice Contentment: Have you ever felt the need to acquire more things constantly? Cultivating gratitude for what you already have can be a powerful antidote. By focusing on the positives in your life, you can reduce the urge to seek out more outside happiness constantly. It is incredible how much more content and fulfilled you can feel when you take the time to appreciate what you already have. Work on cultivating inner happiness and joy.

Avoid Shopping When Emotional: Emotional states can make you more susceptible to persuasive tactics. Avoid making significant purchasing decisions when feeling stressed, sad, or anxious.

Unsubscribe and Opt-Out: Remove yourself from promotional emails and opt out of targeted advertising whenever possible.

Practice Critical Thinking: Analyze claims made in commercials and question whether the product can truly deliver on its promises.

Create a Budget: Allocate specific amounts for different spending categories. Having a budget in place can help prevent impulsive purchases. There are many free online templates that you can download and adapt to your needs. If possible, to hire a financial coach, go for it.

Practice Gratitude: Regularly remind yourself of the things you are grateful for. This can reduce the desire for constant acquisition.

By utilizing these techniques, you can empower yourself to make more deliberate and conscious choices rather than being swayed by commercial influences.

Storytime: The Dance of Glucose Tolerance and Circadian Rhythms

Once upon a time, someone named Glucose lived in a complex city of body cells. Glucose lost memory of the critical role it plays in human existence. Glucose was lost and did not feel important.

Insulin, a hormone secreted by the pancreas, choreographs the body's elegant response to consumed sugars and glucose tolerance.

Glucose learned about glucose tolerance, the body-balanced responses after a meal, effortlessly maintaining blood sugar levels within a harmonious range. However, as with any dance, there were missteps. Insulin resistance, a condition known to disrupt this fluid choreography, could lead to higher blood sugar levels, potentially culminating in the development of type 2 diabetes.

As Glucose got deeper into her quest to find meaning in her life, she unearthed another wondrous connection: the bond between glucose tolerance and the circadian rhythm, the body's internal timekeeper. Like the steady beat of a drum, this rhythm regulated processes over a 24-hour span. She learned that glucose metabolism followed this rhythm, rising and falling in a predictable pattern.

In the early morning, when the world was still draped in a gentle veil of dawn, glucose tolerance was at its zenith. Nevertheless, as the day unfolded its hours, it gradually diminished. Glucose discovered that even the smallest disruptions to this rhythm, like irregular sleep or nighttime feasts, could lead to a discordant tune in glucose tolerance. Shift workers, she realized, were particularly susceptible, their erratic schedules causing a dissonance in their metabolic symphony.

Determined to spread this wisdom, Glucose embarked on a journey to share her insights into the body systems. She advocated for the sanctity of a regular sleep schedule by making the body yawn and alert the body to go to bed. Glucose alerted the body to a headache; there was too much sugar.

Glucose talked to the pancreas trying to compensate for the increase in sugar. With each word she speaks, she illustrates the profound interplay between the body's internal clock and its metabolic processes.

And so, in the heart of that bustling body, Glucose's voice illuminated the path to balanced health. Her tale reminds us that within our bodies lies a dance that can only be truly appreciated when we honor the rhythms that course through our veins. In that dance, we find the essence of life itself, a delicate, ever-changing symphony of health and well-being. The end!

Journaling Time

What information did you find interesting, surprising, and valuable to learn in this chapter?

_____
_____
_____
_____
_____
_____
_____
_____
_____
_____
_____
_____
_____
_____

"You can go far, one step at a time." Solanyi Ulloa

Chapter 6

Physical Activity

Learning Objectives:

- Physical Activity
- Body Systems: Needs for Movement
- Exercise Prescription
- Physical Activity Barriers
- Physical Fitness & Activity (PFA): Shake it, move it, improve it.
- Trial and Error
- The Before, During, and After Physical Activity
- Posture

Hey there! Let's talk about physical activity! Specifically, why do you want to increase yours? Get specific and tell me all about it!

_____

_____

_____

_____

Understanding Physical Activity

As defined by the World Health Organization (WHO), physical activity is any bodily movement that expends energy from skeletal muscles. This includes walking, sports, play, and recreational activities. In this book, I emphasize the term 'physical activity' rather than 'exercise,' although it is important to note that exercise is indeed a form of physical activity. It is a misconception that exercise solely implies rigorous gym routines; in reality, any activity that elevates your heart rate and may induce perspiration qualifies.

Facts and Figures: Astonishingly, around 1.4 billion adults worldwide fall short of engaging in adequate physical activity. Notably, individuals who maintain physical fitness tend to enjoy an extended lifespan of up to seven years compared to their less active counterparts.

Impact on Health: The repercussions of physical inactivity on one's well-being are profound. It heightens the risk of various diseases and diminishes overall quality of life. Cognitive function and a reduction in muscle mass can be adversely affected, paving the way for muscle wasting.

Embracing an active lifestyle promotes longevity and significantly enhances quality of life. By acknowledging the benefits of physical activity and making it an integral part of our daily routines, we embark on a journey toward improved health and overall well-being.

The Vital Role of Exercise-Nurturing Body Systems

The Domino Effect in Your Body: Much like a line of falling dominoes, our body systems are interconnected. A positive change in one area can create a chain reaction of positive effects, while negative behaviors can lead to a series of adverse outcomes. This principle holds true for both our physical and mental well-being. By enhancing one aspect of our health, we initiate a domino effect of positivity. Conversely, engaging in negative behaviors can trigger a cascade of detrimental consequences within our body systems, potentially culminating in disease.

The Significance of Physical Activity: Regular physical activity significantly reduces the risk of various ailments, including heart diseases, hypertension, diabetes, and several forms of cancer. It plays a pivotal role in enhancing the performance of our body systems, contributing to an overall sense of well-being and a more appealing physical appearance.

A Holistic Approach to Health: Numerous studies affirms the benefits of physical activity for both body and mind. Regular physical activity promotes the growth of bone mass, boosts flexibility, stability, and muscle strength, and even lowers the risk of injuries. By embracing a lifestyle that incorporates regular physical activity, we invest in the holistic well-being of our body systems, setting the stage for a healthier, happier life.

Behavioral Acquired Diseases (BAD): Taking Charge of Your Health Behavioral Acquired Diseases (BAD) are health conditions attributed to individual choices, decisions, and lifestyles. This category has a range of ailments, including type 2 diabetes, high blood pressure, atherosclerosis (hardening of the arteries), strokes, kidney disease, various forms of cancer, pulmonary diseases, and more. The critical factor in BADs is that they often result from habits and behaviors that an individual adopts, making them largely preventable through positive lifestyle changes.

Understanding the Root Causes: BADs find their roots in specific habits and lifestyle choices that individuals make. These include inadequate physical activity, smoking, excessive alcohol consumption, poor dietary habits, irregular eating patterns, and illicit drug use, among others. Recognizing these patterns is the first step towards proactively preventing and managing these conditions.

Empowering Change for a Healthier Future: While BADs may be prevalent today, they can be prevented. By acknowledging the impact of our choices on our health, we gain the power to make positive changes. Engaging in regular physical activity, adopting a balanced diet, and avoiding harmful substances like tobacco and excessive alcohol are pivotal steps. Through informed decisions and conscious efforts, we can break free from the clutches of BADs and pave the way for a brighter and healthier future.

Neurological: Scientific studies have shown how the lack of physical activity negatively impacts the brain and increases risks for diseases such as Parkinson's disease, Alzheimer's disease, different types of dementias, Multiple Sclerosis, Strokes, and Mini strokes, to name a few. I have been working with patients with the above conditions for over 15 years and patients with many other neurological issues, and I cannot help but feel sad many times with the cognitive decline these patients suffer and seeing how these diseases advance. If you or a loved one has had any of these conditions, you know what I am talking about; if you are unfamiliar, it is ok whenever you can do a brief internet search on them.

Engaging in regular physical activity brings a multitude of benefits. It enhances mental awareness, leading to sharper cognitive functions. This active lifestyle promotes better sleep quality, heightens attention levels, and improves concentration. With increased retention capabilities, information is absorbed more effectively. Moreover, it boosts motivation and reduces anxiety, contributing to better mood stabilization. Physical activity is a powerful stress reducer, providing a sense of calm and alleviating fatigue. Notably, it also plays a role in lowering the risk of developing dementia, underlining its profound impact on long-term cognitive health.

Regular physical activity triggers a cascade of "feel-good" hormones, commonly known as the DOSE effect—dopamine, oxytocin, serotonin, and endorphins. This physiological response leads to increased happiness, elevated moods, and overall well-being. Extensive scientific research supports the notion that individuals who incorporate exercise into their routines often experience reduced symptoms of depression and enjoy enhanced mental health. The positive impact of physical activity on emotional well-being is a powerful testament to its holistic benefits.

Cardiovascular Health and Physical Activity

Poor cardiovascular health, often associated with insufficient physical fitness, can lead to weakened heart muscles, elevated levels of harmful cholesterol, an increased risk of arrhythmias, reduced blood circulation, and a higher likelihood of experiencing muscle cramps. On the flip side, embracing regular physical activity brings a wealth of benefits to your cardiovascular system. It strengthens the heart muscles, as well as the arteries and veins, while also reinforcing levels of beneficial cholesterol. This improves blood flow, ensuring better nourishment for your organs and tissues. Moreover, engaging in physical activity is a powerful tool in reducing high blood pressure and heart attack risk. Taking care of your heart through regular physical activity yields many positive outcomes.

Fortunately, many cardiovascular diseases can be prevented, or their onset delayed by increasing physical activity. Your heart serves as your body's engine, and a strong heart translates to a stronger, more resilient you.

Respiratory System

As a nursing intern, I was privileged to work in the labor and delivery unit, where I witnessed multiple successful childbirths. The experience left an indelible mark on me as I watched the commencement of life outside the womb. Witnessing the newborn's first breath, observing the tiny chest and diaphragm at work, and hearing the resounding cry filling the room was magnificent. This cry also served as one of the earliest indicators of the newborn's lung health. The lungs are magnificent organs that enable the very breath of life, and it is crucial to maintain their health.

Respiratory health is of utmost importance, and poor respiratory health stemming from insufficient physical activity can lead to elevated susceptibility to respiratory infections, diminished tidal volume, and, subsequently, reduced oxygen levels. This can directly impact cognitive functions, resulting in impaired decision-making and decreased mental acuity. On the other hand, regular physical activity can help fortify respiratory muscles, amplify tidal volume, heighten mental alertness, and significantly reduce the incidence of respiratory infections such as sinus infections, common colds, and flu cases.

Let us take a moment to appreciate the lungs for the gift of the breath of life they provide. By taking slow, deep breaths, we can bring attention to the sensation of air entering our nose, expanding our chest, abdomen, and shoulders, and then the calmness and warmth of the air leaving our mouth. Regular physical activity and deep breathing exercises can help maintain healthy respiratory function and provide many positive outcomes.

Digestive System

Decreased physical activity can reduce gut microbiome, which are the beneficial bacteria essential for a robust immune system. Additionally, it can lead to decreased digestion and increased occurrences of constipation. An imbalance in the digestive microbiome has been associated with various health concerns, including obesity, heart disease, diabetes, as well as digestive disorders like irritable bowel syndrome (IBS), gastroenteritis, ulcerative colitis, diverticulosis, and many others.

On the other hand, embracing an active lifestyle has numerous positive effects on digestion. This encompasses an enhanced metabolism, fortifying the immune system, and a healthier gut microbiome with reduced inflammation. Moreover, it leads to heightened energy levels, aids in preventing gallstones, and significantly reduces the risk of colon cancer.

Urinary System

Decreased physical activity can lead to various negative outcomes for urinary health. This includes an elevated risk of kidney disease, high blood pressure, body fluid imbalance, and a higher likelihood of developing kidney stones and infections. Additionally, it increases the risk of urinary stress incontinence.

Conversely, engaging in regular physical activity brings about a host of positive effects on urinary health. This includes strengthening pelvic floor muscles, resulting in a stronger bladder and fewer nighttime bathroom trips. Furthermore, increased blood filtration enhances the immune system by removing more toxins and waste products from the body. This contributes to a healthier urinary system and significantly decreases urinary tract infections.

Musculoskeletal System

When physical activity is lacking, it can lead to a range of adverse outcomes for muscular and skeletal health. This includes decreased muscle tone, strength, and lower bone density, which increases the risk of fractures and injuries. It can leave you feeling drained and lacking vitality.

On the flip side, increased physical activity has many positive effects on muscular and skeletal health. It boosts energy levels, enabling you to accomplish more tasks and activities. Moreover, it leads to stronger muscles and bones, providing a foundation for a stronger, more resilient you. This, in turn, reduces the risk of falls and related injuries while also preventing conditions like osteoporosis. Increased physical activity also diminishes chronic pain, enhances mobility, and sharpens reflexes.

Endocrine System

The endocrine system, a network of glands that produce and regulate hormones, plays a crucial role in how physical activity impacts the body. Our body releases hormones that help regulate various physiological functions when we engage in physical activity. For instance, Growth Hormone, stimulated by physical activity, aids tissue repair and muscle growth. Physical activity also influences thyroid hormones, affecting metabolism and energy levels. Regular physical activity can also help regulate blood sugar levels, reducing the risk of insulin-related conditions like diabetes. Moreover, exercise supports the release of endorphins, often called "feel-good" hormones, which improve mood and reduce stress levels.

Regular physical activity plays a pivotal role in maintaining hormonal balance within the body. When physical activity levels decrease, it can lead to a decrease in hormone levels, potentially causing homeostasis issues and hormonal disorders. Moreover, a sedentary lifestyle may inadvertently promote the growth and reproduction of cancer cells, making it crucial to stay active. Inactivity also elevates cortisol levels, contributing to elevated stress levels and associated health problems. This includes an increased risk of developing chronic conditions like diabetes and hyper/hypothyroidism.

Conversely, engaging in regular physical activity yields a multitude of positive hormonal outcomes. Studies have shown a reduced risk of colon and rectal cancer in physically active individuals. Additionally, increased physical activity can lower the risks associated with certain types of cancer. Exercise positively impacts hormones like dopamine, known for its stress-reducing and mood-enhancing effects, and serotonin, which supports sleep quality, mood regulation, digestion, memory, and sexual well-being. Furthermore, physical activity contributes to more effective regulation of testosterone and estrogen levels.

Integumentary System

When physical activity levels decrease, hormone levels also decrease, potentially causing homeostasis and hormonal disorders. Moreover, a sedentary lifestyle may inadvertently promote the growth and reproduction of cancer cells. Making it crucial to stay active. Inactivity also elevates cortisol levels, contributing to heightened stress and associated health problems. This includes an increased risk of developing chronic conditions like diabetes and hyper/hypothyroidism.

Conversely, engaging in regular physical activity yields a multitude of positive hormonal outcomes. Studies have shown a reduced risk of colon and rectal cancer in physically active individuals. Additionally, increased physical activity can lower the risks associated with certain types of cancer. Physical activity positively impacts hormones like dopamine, known for its stress-reducing and mood-enhancing effects, and serotonin, which supports sleep quality, mood regulation, digestion, memory, and sexual well-being. Furthermore, physical activity contributes to more effective regulation of testosterone and estrogen levels.

Health On Demand Nurturing the Universe Within

Problem: Vigorous physical activity without a structured workout routine can worsen existing skin conditions.

Solution: It is essential to establish a pre- and post-workout skincare routine.

Physical Activity Recommendation by the World Health Organization (WHO) as of 2023

Infants (<1 year old): Engage in floor-based play. For those not yet crawling, spend at least 30 minutes lying on their stomach with adult supervision, spread throughout the day.

Kids (1-4 years old): Aim for at least 3 hours of exercise daily, with one-hour intervals in the morning, midday, and afternoon. Avoid restraining them for over 1 hour (e.g., prams, highchairs, carriers).

Children and Adolescents (5–17 years old): Strive for at least 60 minutes of moderate to vigorous physical activity.

Adults (18-64 years old): Target an average of 150-300 minutes of moderate-intensity physical activity per week or at least 75 minutes of vigorous activities.

Older Adults (>65 years old): It is the same as adults, emphasizing exercises that enhance strength and balance to prevent falls and muscle wasting.

Pregnant and Postpartum Women (without complications): Aim for a minimum of 150 minutes of light-to-moderate intensity physical activity to reduce risks like pre-eclampsia, gestational diabetes, delivery complications, and postpartum depression and to prevent excess gestational weight.

Even 30 minutes of physical activity 2-3 times a week is a positive start.

Physical Activity Barriers

Physical activity barriers can present themselves in various forms, making it challenging for individuals to engage in regular physical activity.

Lack of Motivation: Finding the drive and enthusiasm to engage in physical activity can be a struggle for many. It is essential to discover activities that genuinely interest and inspire you. It is challenging for individuals to engage in regular physical activity.

Lack of Energy: Fatigue or low energy levels can deter individuals from participating in physical activities. Implementing a sleep schedule, a balanced diet, and maintaining proper hydration can significantly improve energy levels.

Lack of Time: Busy schedules and demanding responsibilities often leave little time for dedicated physical activity. However, even short bursts of physical activity can contribute to overall fitness. Task management and prioritization can carve out space for physical activity.

Lack of Appropriate Environment: Environmental factors like extreme temperatures or unfavorable weather conditions can make outdoor activities less appealing. Having alternatives for indoor exercise, such as home workouts or gym access, can help circumvent this barrier.

Physical Limitations: Existing health conditions or physical limitations may restrict certain types of activities. It is crucial to choose a physical activity that aligns with your abilities.

Lack of Social Support: A lack of encouragement or companionship in physical activities can dampen motivation. Joining group classes or finding reliable workout buddies can provide the necessary support and accountability.

Fear of Injury: Concerns about getting injured during physical activity can be a significant deterrent. Engaging in proper warm-ups, utilizing appropriate equipment, and seeking guidance from fitness professionals can help mitigate this fear.

Monotony and Boredom: Performing the same physical activity can lead to monotony and boredom. Exploring various activities, from dancing to hiking, can add excitement and variety to your routine.

Financial Constraints: The cost of gym memberships, fitness classes, or specialized equipment can be a significant barrier. However, various budget-friendly options are available, including outdoor activities and home workouts.

By identifying and addressing these barriers, individuals can take proactive steps toward overcoming challenges and establishing a sustainable, enjoyable, and adequate physical activity routine. Celebrate every small step towards greatness!

Which challenges are preventing you from engaging in physical activities?

_____
_____
_____

How can you overcome these challenges?

_____
_____
_____
_____

Activities to Consider

- Pleasure Walking (around nature even better)
- Dancing
- Using stairs
- Gardening
- Yard Work
- Housework such as swiping and mopping.
- Home Exercise

- Gym Exercise
- Brisk Walking
- Rope Jumping
- Running
- Swimming
- Bicycling

Fitness classes encompass a wide range of activities, each offering unique benefits. From the tranquility of Yoga and the rhythmic movements of Zumba to the core-strengthening focus of Pilates and the high-intensity intervals of HIIT, there is a class to suit every preference. Kickboxing and strength training provides dynamic, empowering workouts while cycling and treadmill sessions offer practical cardiovascular training. Rowing and water aerobics provide excellent alternatives for those seeking a low-impact option. The diverse fitness classes ensure something for everyone, catering to various fitness levels and interests.

If you lean towards more intense activities, there is a range of rough-and-tumble exercises and sports. This includes disciplines like Wing Chun, Kung Fu, Jiu-Jitsu, Brazilian Jiu-Jitsu, Karate, Muay Thai (Thai Boxing), Boxing, and Jeet Kune Do (the martial art founded by Bruce Lee). You might wonder why I am bringing these up. Well, in my teenage years, I used to take Karate classes, and truthfully, it significantly contributed to my discipline and mental fortitude and helped reduce my anxiety and stress levels along the way.

Trial and Error

We all go through the same stages when learning something; the same holds true for physical activity. At the Basic Level, it is about those initial attempts. Then comes the Intermediate stage when we have achieved a satisfactory level. Finally, we reach the Advanced stage, were repetition and practice lead to proficiency.

So, here is a little recommendation: the next time you catch yourself saying, "I am not good at this or that," hold your horses, honey! Take a step back and reflect on how many times you have attempted it. If you can count or even remember the number of tries, guess what? You need to try more. We all have the internal capacity to reach an advanced level in anything we set our minds.

Give it a fair shot when trying different physical activity routines or fitness classes. Try it at least five times before deciding if it is the right fit for you. I remember my first time in a Yoga, cycling, and Zumba class. I felt like I was stumbling through, embarrassed and unsure. My primitive brain was busy comparing me to everyone else in the room. I was fixated on their grace and poise while I was still figuring things out on my very first try! Later, I realized it did not serve me to compare. Each person is on a unique journey, even if we share similar goals.

Moreover, remember those in the classroom who had attended those classes for a while. No wonder they knew the steps like the back of their hand! It all makes sense now.

Before Physical Activity:

- Prioritize your sleep to ensure you have the energy for your workout.
- Hydrate with plain water (naturally flavored water is okay) and avoid sugary beverages.
- Set a specific time for exercise and establish your goals.
- Plan your next meal after your pre-workout routine.
- Create a motivating music playlist.
- Wash your hands.
- If you are prone to acne or skin issues, I recommend cleansing your face with a gentle, organic cleanser with as few added chemicals as possible.
- Avoid makeup if possible.

- Apply a thin layer of skin moisturizer with organic ingredients to allow your pores to breathe and facilitate sweat removal from your body.
- Wash your hands.
- Hydrate, hydrate, hydrate with plain water (naturally flavored water is okay) and avoid sugary beverages. I cannot stress this enough.
- Remember to protect your skin from prolonged sun exposure when working outside. Choose mornings and evenings for outdoor workouts, as the sun's UV rays are less damaging during those hours.
- If possible, avoid midday sun exposure at all costs.
- Stretch before starting any physical activity. It provides a nice warm-up for your muscles, bones, and ligaments, signaling your body, "Hey! It's time to work out; let's get it done!"
- Ensure your environment is free from any safety hazards.
- If necessary, have a small nutritional snack, but avoid exercising immediately after eating hefty meals.
- Wear comfortable clothing and shoes.
- Have a hand towel on your hand to dry sweat. Microfiber eco-friendly are good options for many people, as they tend to be gentle on the skin.

During Physical Activity

Breathing and Sweating: Pay attention to your breath when performing a physical activity. Take deep, intentional breaths. As you sweat, think of it as your body shedding the excess and letting go. Embrace the process, knowing that you're making positive changes. Take deep breaths in and out, and if you are sweating, let that fat cry and enjoy it.

Hydration Importance: Hydration must be stressed more. It's vital for your body's functions, especially during physical activity. Water helps regulate your temperature, lubricates joints, and carries nutrients to cells. Keep replenishing to ensure your body operates at its best.

Mindful Presence: Engage fully in your workout. Let it be a non-negotiable part of your routine. Be in the moment, feel the movements, and embrace the activity. Let go of thoughts about the past or future. This mindful approach enhances your physical engagement and provides mental clarity and focus.

Listening to Your Body: Understand your body's signals. If it's asking for a break, slow down or rest. If it signals that it's time to stop, heed that message. This awareness is crucial in avoiding overexertion or pushing past your limits, which can lead to injuries.

Breathing and Fat Burning: When you burn fat, it's transformed into carbon dioxide. This combines with the water in your body and is expelled through various bodily fluids like urine, sweat, and even feces. Appreciate this natural process of your body working to become physically and mentally healthier.

After your Physical Activity

Hydration: Replenish lost fluids by drinking water. This helps restore your body's balance and aids in the recovery process.

Stretching: Allocate 5-10 minutes for stretching exercises. This promotes flexibility, reduces muscle tension, and prevents stiffness.

Personal Care: Take a refreshing shower to cleanse and cool down. Change into clean underwear, socks, and dry clothes to ensure comfort and hygiene.

Skin Care: Moisturize your skin to replenish moisture lost during the workout. This helps maintain skin health and prevents dryness.

Nutritious Refueling: If you're hungry, opt for nutritious options. Focus on replenishing protein and carbohydrates to support muscle recovery. Consider options like a protein shake, a piece of fruit, or a balanced meal.

7 Strategies to Optimize Your Health & Prevent Chronic Illnesses.

Note: Post-workout care is crucial for maximizing the benefits of your exercise routine and ensuring your body recovers effectively.

The When of Physical Activity

Shake it, move it, improve it. Now, if you're anything like me, a self-proclaimed busybee, you know the struggle. During the COVID-19 pandemic, I bid farewell to the gym and my regular workouts. The days got packed with caring for family, friends, patients, and their families, leaving little room for me. My exercise routine was replaced by running around like a chicken without a head, as I was needed in multiple places simultaneously. I also found myself lifting corpses with my team to carry them on stretchers and bring them outside to the morticians, as they were not allowed in the buildings due to the lockdown.

Life's demands piled up, and finding time for physical activity became a challenge amidst it all. Time, energy, and motivation seemed in short supply. The gym, once my sanctuary, vanished from my routine. My warm-ups, diverse exercise routines, and faithful attendance to fitness classes became memories. I turned to sporadic hikes in their absence, but even that faded, resulting in a 20-pound weight gain. The last time I carried this much weight was during a pregnancy complicated by pre-eclampsia and near-gestational diabetes. Fast forward to today, and physical activity is non-negotiable in my calendar. The journey back wasn't smooth, but I persisted, recalling the post-workout high. The inevitable soreness tested my resolve, but after a week, I tried again. I advise starting slow—small steps in the right direction beat giant leaps followed by setbacks. I carve out 10-minute high-intensity sessions each week. Once it's on my calendar, excuses dissolve. When my mind toys with "I'm too tired" or "I don't have time" games, logic steps in: "Really, GIRL!!! Ten minutes for the most important thing on your calendar!!" And just like that, I'm committed, often ending up with 37-40 minutes of refreshing physical activity!

The Most important thing is to create an unbreakable movement/physical activity routine. For example, my physical activity routine kicks in after a long and stressful workday.

Good Body Posture

Did you know that maintaining good posture can do wonders for your body and mind? Not only does it help you appear confident, but it also:

Reduced pain: Good posture can help reduce pain in the neck, back, shoulders, and other body areas; this is because it helps to align the spine and other bones in the body, which can reduce strain on muscles and joints.

Improved breathing: Good posture can help to improve breathing by opening the airways and allowing more air to flow into the lungs, which is helpful for people with respiratory problems, such as asthma or COPD.

Increased energy: Good posture can improve energy levels by making it easier to move around and breathe, and it takes less effort to move when the body is aligned correctly.

Improved confidence: Good posture can help to improve confidence by making you look and feel more confident because it gives off an air of authority and power.

Reduced stress: Good posture can help reduce stress by making you feel more relaxed and in control. It also helps to reduce muscle tension and improve circulation.

Tips for improving your body posture

Stand up straight: When you are standing, make sure to keep your shoulders back and your head up. Your ears should align with your shoulders, and your chin should parallel the ground.

Sit up straight: When you are sitting, keep your back straight and your shoulders back. Your feet should be flat on the floor, and your knees should be bent at a 90-degree angle.

Be aware of your posture throughout the day: Knowing your posture throughout the day and adjusting as needed is important to help you maintain good posture even when not thinking about it.

Strengthen your core muscles: Strong core muscles can help to support your spine and improve your posture. You can do several exercises to strengthen your core muscles, such as planks, crunches, and leg lifts.

Get regular physical activity: This can help improve your overall fitness and flexibility, leading to better posture.

If you struggle to improve your body posture, consider seeing a physical therapist or an experienced and well-trained neurology-based chiropractor. They can help you identify any underlying problems contributing to your poor posture and create a personalized plan to help you improve it.

Journaling Time

What information did you find interesting, surprising, and valuable to learn in this chapter?

_____

_____

_____

_____

_____

_____

_____

_____

_____

_____

_____

_____

_____

'Growth' and 'progress' are among the keywords in our vocabulary. But modern man now carries Strontium 90 in his bones... DDT in his fat, asbestos in his lungs. A little more on this 'progress' and 'growth' and this man will be dead"- Morris K. "Mo" Udall

Chapter 7

Avoiding Harmful Chemicals: A Journey Back to Basics

In this industrialized society, we want everything faster, cheaper, and better. Unfortunately, nature does not work like that. Yet humans have found a way to meet the demand for faster and cheaper, even if it's not necessarily better. However, this comes with a price tag that is too high for our bodies, especially when it comes to products we consume daily, such as food, personal hygiene products, and the chemicals we use to clean our environment.

Back to Basics (BTB): More than 4,000 substances can be added to food, and approximately 350,000 artificial chemicals (human-made). For your sake and mine, I will discuss the most relevant chemicals commonly used as of 2023.

Understanding Preservatives and Additives: Preservatives are considered additives, but when it comes to additives, not all are preservatives. Don't worry if you need clarification; I have got you covered. Additives can be organic and non-organic (Genetically Modified Organisms, also called GMOs),

Food preservatives limit the growth of microbes that can cause illness. These preservatives provide a product with a longer shelf life, improved taste, and a better appearance. However, the problem is this: the longer the shelf life, the longer the list of preservatives, and the less nutritional value.

Nitrates can be naturally found in plants like leafy greens, beets, and celery. They can also be synthetically produced as sodium nitrate or sodium nitrite. When we consume nitrates from plants, our bodies effectively convert them to benefit our cells, improving heart health and reducing inflammation due to their antioxidant properties. However, when we ingest nitrates from synthetic sources, the body converts them into nitrosamines, which have been linked to various cancers, including those of the lungs, brain, liver, kidney, bladder, stomach, gastrointestinal tract, and colorectal area. Chemical nitrates are present in cured meats like hot dogs, cold cuts, bacon, and other processed meats. Additionally, nitrosamine compounds can be found in certain medications used for conditions like diabetes, acid reflux, elevated blood pressure, and heartburn. These medications may include but are not limited to, ranitidine, nizatidine, metformin, and angiotensin II receptor blockers (ARBs).

Back to Basics (BTB): Most medications are essential in managing health issues; they provide necessary support. However, it's crucial to remember that they don't offer a cure. They're akin to applying a band-aid to an infected wound; the band-aid needs regular replacement, and if further steps are not taken to heal the injury, a bandage will always be necessary. On the other hand, acting means addressing the root problem, allowing you to discontinue the medication.

I take great pride in my patients who have followed my guidance. They have effectively managed chronic conditions and often reduced their daily medication intake with proper support from their primary healthcare provider. Unfortunately, those who didn't heed my advice, well, some are no longer with us because of disease complications. In contrast, others now rely on a regimen of 10-25 pills daily, not to mention complications of their chronic illnesses.

Ultimately, your body is the most trustworthy authority. It possesses the wisdom to discern what's beneficial and what's detrimental. Through this book, I hope you learn to attune to your body's signals and make decisions that align with your unique needs.

Food Coloring

Color is an influential factor in enhancing the appeal of food and various products. However, it's regrettable that most food colorings in today's products are heavily processed and synthetically derived. These chemical compounds can be detrimental to your health, potentially leading to a range of issues, including cancer, behavioral disorders, and even depression.

It is advisable to steer clear of foods containing artificial coloring, particularly those with the following additives:

- Red Dye Number 3
- Red 40
- Blue #1
- Blue #2
- Yellow #5
- Yellow #6
- Natural Green Color

Many food products contain artificial food coloring to improve their appearance and make them more attractive to consumers. However, it's essential to understand that these additives negatively affect health. Studies have linked them to an increased risk of cancer, behavioral problems (especially in children), hyperactivity, allergies, migraines, and various mental disorders. Therefore, it is crucial to be aware of the potential risks associated with consuming products that contain artificial food coloring and to choose healthier alternatives whenever possible.

Alternative and Health*er* Food Coloring: Turmeric is very potent, and you will thank me later if you choose a pan strictly for recipes where you will use turmeric as a food coloring. Organic powders extracted from blueberries, raspberries, carrots, beets, purple cabbage, and matcha powder. If you search the internet for "How to make Natural and Organic Food Coloring," you will find many ways. (You're so welcome ☺).

MSG (Monosodium Glutamate): A prevalent food allergen and flavor enhancer, finds widespread use in various products worldwide, with prominence in the U.S. It is added to restaurant dishes, fast food, frozen meals, canned soups, and salty snacks to increase their taste. However, MSG poses significant risks to both human and animal health. Its consumption has been linked to a range of health issues, including headaches, numbness, obesity, disruptions in the brain and nervous system, gastrointestinal problems, reproductive issues, and high blood pressure, among others.

High Fructose Corn Syrup: A prevalent sweetener in many processed foods, has been linked to many health issues. These range from diabetes and weight gain to obesity, liver disease, heart problems, and even cancer. Additionally, its consumption has been associated with gout, chronic inflammation, and numerous other health concerns. Given these potential risks, it's advisable to exercise caution when consuming products containing this sweetener. Exploring alternative options for sweetening foods and beverages can contribute to a more balanced and healthful diet, reducing the likelihood of encountering these associated health problems. Avoid products containing this sweetener at all costs if possible.

Silica: Also known as silicon, silicon dioxide, or E 551, is a toxic chemical to the human body. Studies have indicated a link between silica exposure and various health issues, including an increased risk of cancer, immune system suppression leading to more infections, and urinary and respiratory problems. It is crucial to be aware of the potential dangers associated with this chemical compound.

Lecithin: Is a group of chemicals naturally present in certain foods and animals. It is widely utilized as a food additive and in cosmetics, medications, and supplements, with soy lecithin being a common variant. However, it's important to note that soy lecithin can have various effects on the body, including potential weight gain, dizziness, blurred vision, rashes, decreased appetite, nausea, vomiting, and low blood pressure. If you use products containing soy lecithin or its derivatives, exercise caution and be attentive to how your body responds before, during, and after use.

Guar Gum: A versatile substance added to a wide range of products, including beverages, dairy items, processed cheeses, baked goods, processed meats, cereals, vegetable juices, soups, sauces, salad dressings, puddings, medications, textiles, paper, and cosmetics. While some studies suggest positive effects when used moderately, it's important to note that this chemical can also lead to allergic reactions in specific individuals and may cause symptoms such as gas, bloating, and digestive disruptions.

Xatham Gum: Chemical additives to food, beverages, personal care products, low-fat foods, syrups, salad dressing, alcohol, ice creams, baked goods, unique care products, and industrial products. Even though this chemical is considered "safe," it can cause flatulence, bloating, flu-like symptoms, and respiratory system issues.

Refined Salt (Iodized Salt): Refined salt, commonly known as iodized salt, undergoes mechanical and chemical processes during its harvesting, which leads to the removal of essential minerals. It's worth noting that many salt mines are situated in polluted environments. This type of salt can potentially be toxic to the human body. It can bind with vital minerals in your body, leading to their excretion and rendering your system more vulnerable to illnesses. Additionally, numerous salt companies incorporate chemicals like sulfuric acid, chlorine, aluminum silicate, dextrose, and other harmful substances to human health. The amount of iodine in refined salt is insufficient for preventing thyroid issues. Consider opting for un-refined salt unless you have any medical contraindications. Un-refined salt may contain all the elements necessary to sustain Prana, the life-giving force. Here are some alternatives to refined salt:

219

- Mediterranean Sea Salt: A healthier option compared to table salt.
- Celtic Sea Salt: Harvested in the same way as ancient Celts did over 2,000 years ago.
- Un-refined Redmond Salt: Harvested from salt deposits near Redmond in Utah.
- Pink Salt: While not extensively researched, some studies suggest that the health benefits of pink salt may not be as significant for the human body as table salt. It's important to note that some unscrupulous manufacturers use dynamite to access pink salt, which can result in explosive materials becoming attached to the salt. As a rule of thumb, choose reputable brands, as not all pink salt is the same.
- Kala Namak (Himalayan Black Salt): Known to have antioxidant properties.
- Black Lava Salt: Harvested from the coasts of Cyprus and Hawaii, this type of salt is created by incorporating activated charcoal from the local lava. Activated charcoal is believed to help detoxify the body from impurities, but scientific data supporting this claim is limited.

In conclusion, using un-refined salts in moderation is advisable, and steer clear of refined salts.

Refined Sugar

Sugar is a carbohydrate that the body converts into glucose, which serves as fuel. Unfortunately, refined sugar is added to a wide range of products, from food and beverages to desserts and many other items. High sugar intake can be addictive and lead to diabetes, obesity, weight gain, heart disease, and metabolic syndrome, among others.

Whenever possible choose products without added sugar and consider natural sugars found in fruits and vegetables whenever possible. When reading food labels, pay close attention to sugars, added sugars, and carbohydrates (as carbs ultimately convert into sugar, specifically glucose). Honey, agave syrup, stevia, monk fruit, dates, yacon syrup, and maple syrup are all viable options to sweeten your food and beverages without consuming refined sugar. Each of these alternatives offers its unique flavor profile and may have specific health benefits, so it's worth exploring which ones work best for your taste and dietary preferences. Remember, even though these alternatives may have some nutritional advantages, consuming them mindfully is essential as part of a balanced diet.

Sugar alcohols like erythritol, maltitol, xylitol, and others are commonly used as alternatives to sugar. However, it's important to note that these substitutes sometimes have more negative effects than sugar. They have been associated with stomach issues, toxicity concerns, and hormonal disruptions, as the body may struggle to digest or absorb some of these compounds. It's advisable to be cautious when using sugar alcohols in your diet.

Aspartame is an artificial sweetener approximately 200 times sweeter than regular sugar. It is found in sugar-free beverages, jelly, Kool-Aid, and supplements. However, it is considered toxic to humans and can lead to various adverse effects. Due to its rapid impact on blood glucose levels, aspartame has been associated with increased anxiety and can negatively impact the pancreas. It is essential to be mindful of its consumption.

BHA (Butylated hydroxyanisole) and BHT (Butylated hydroxytoluene) are found in products like potato chips, cereals, chewing gums, and vegetable oils. However, they have been associated with concerning health effects. These additives can potentially alter brain function, leading to behavioral issues, and have even been linked to cancer. It's important to be aware of their presence in our products.

Trans Fats Trans fats are unsaturated fats that undergo hydrogenation, turning liquid oils into solid fats. They are commonly found in processed foods like fried items, baked goods, and packaged snacks. Artificial trans fats, produced through hydrogenation, have been linked to heart disease. They raise "bad" LDL cholesterol and lower "good" HDL cholesterol levels. Many health organizations advise limiting their consumption, leading to regulations in various regions to restrict their use in food production.

Titanium Dioxide (TiO2) is a common additive in various products, including personal care items like pressed powders, lotions, and sunscreens, as well as paints, ceramics, and textiles. While TiO2 has been associated with cancer, studies indicate that this risk primarily arises from inhalation rather than skin contact. To err on the side of caution, consider opting for cosmetics with more straightforward ingredient lists and less harmful chemicals.

Phthalates are found in hundreds of products, such as personal care products, toys, daily-use containers, and medical tubing, and are added to many types of plastic to make them last longer. Phthalates cause endocrine disruptions (hormonal issues) in adults, kids, and youth, and of course, I am sure the elderly population is not exempt from their risks, which include fertility issues affecting child growth and development. Many countries have restricted the use of phthalates to reduce health risks.

Alternative: Glass containers with silicone lids that are non-toxic and plastic-free, covers made of safer choices such as acacia wood.

PFAS (per- and polyfluoroalkyl substances), including **PFOS (perfluorooctane sulfonic acid)** and **PFOA (perfluorooctanoic acid**) are prevalent in various products like food packaging, clothing, and non-stick cookware. Their persistence is concerning, leading to bioaccumulation in wildlife and potential environmental contamination. Animal studies have revealed exposure to high levels of these chemicals results in a range of health issues, including reproductive, liver, immune system, thyroid, and growth complications. While the full extent of their impact on human health remains uncertain, their known toxicity levels suggest potential harm.

Brominated Vegetable Oil (BVO) is a food additive used to preserve fruit flavors in certain products. It can potentially harm human health and has been banned in Japan and Europe.

Potassium Bromate is a food additive known to be a cancer-causing agent. Studies in animals have concluded that it causes kidney, thyroid, and gastrointestinal cancer. Given its carcinogenic effects in animals, there is an increased likelihood that humans may develop the same types of cancer. It's crucial to read the ingredient list of products carefully and avoid those containing potassium bromate.

Propyl Paraben is a chemical commonly used as a preservative in food, personal care products, and pharmaceuticals. However, parabens and their derivatives have been linked to hormone disruption, cancer, allergies, and reproductive problems. To minimize exposure to this compound, it's advisable to choose products that are labeled as paraben-free.

Glyphosate is a widely used herbicide employed to eliminate unwanted weeds and grasses commonly found in agricultural and gardening practices. The issue arises when residues of this chemical are detected in various fruits and vegetables. Although some studies suggest it may not pose significant harm to human health, it's important to approach these findings with caution. As a precaution, opting for organic products whenever possible is advisable. This chemical may potentially affect foods like lentils, oats, beans, chickpeas, canola, corn, cotton, soybeans, wheat, and sugar beets.

Aflatoxins are naturally occurring toxins found in crops like corn, peanuts, tree nuts, and even cow's milk if the cow has consumed contaminated food. The contamination can occur during harvesting or storage. While inhalation exposure is rare, it can happen when handling contaminated crops. However, the most common exposure route is consuming contaminated foods. Aflatoxins are associated with an increased risk of liver cancer. To minimize exposure to this toxin, buy organic food as often as possible. Pay close attention to expiration dates on all your products, especially peanuts, peanut butter, and nut butter, and discard products that look moldy, shriveled, or discolored.

Aristolochic Acid is a naturally occurring compound found in many plants. Some herbal products use these plants to address symptoms like gout, arthritis, and inflammation. However, it's crucial to check supplement labels for aristolochic Acid and avoid products containing it.

This Acid has been associated with cancers of the upper urinary tract and bladder, as well as kidney damage. Be aware that unscrupulous manufacturers might use alternative names to disguise their presence. It's advisable to opt for products with fewer ingredients and carefully research each one, a practice I follow.

Benzene is a chemical found both in nature and can be synthetically produced. In the U.S., it ranks as the 20th most used chemical. It's highly flammable and can be present in various sources, including cigarette smoke, crude oil, and gasoline. Benzene is also found in lubricants, detergents, pesticides, dyes, drugs, plastics, synthetic fibers, and resins. Exposure to Benzene can occur through secondhand smoke (which can be more harmful than direct smoking), glues, detergents, paints, and even well water. Benzene disrupts cellular function, potentially leading to anemia, weakened immune system, bone problems, irregular menstrual cycles, male infertility, and fetal abnormalities. Furthermore, it's a known carcinogen, with Leukemia being the most common cancer associated with it in both humans and animals. Benzene is also referred to by other names such as aniline, cyclohexa-1,3,5-triene, and phenol. It's important to note that products like antiperspirants, deodorants, and body sprays from approximately 54% of all brands may contain Benzene. It is recommended to opt for products with organic formulations whenever possible.

Benzo[a]pyrene is a hazardous chemical known to be carcinogenic and poses risks of poisoning. It can also cause harm to a developing fetus and negatively affect both male and female reproductive systems. Exposure to this chemical can lead to bronchitis, skin rashes, and the formation of warts. Unfortunately, benzo[a]pyrene is present in various sources, including coal, cigarette smoke (a solid reason to avoid smoking), grilled foods, wood smoke, gas products, water, and soil. It's crucial to be aware of these potential sources to minimize exposure.

Ethylene Oxide is a known carcinogenic substance, meaning it has the potential to cause cancer. It has been associated with various types of cancer, including lymphoma, leukemia, stomach cancer, and breast cancer. Exposure to this harmful compound can occur through inhalation or ingestion. It is essential to be aware that ethylene oxide can be present in a range of products and settings, including detergents, pharmaceuticals, textiles, adhesives, cosmetics, and certain solvents like water, ethanol, acetone, and methanol, and it may even be found in some surgical equipment. Taking precautions to limit exposure to this chemical is essential for safeguarding health.

BTB (Back to Basics): The impact of certain chemicals goes beyond just the individual exposed; it can also affect future generations. Research has revealed alterations in DNA patterns that are passed down through offspring. These changes have been associated not only with genetic diseases, but it's worth considering that this issue may be a consequence of the dietary choices made by our grandparents. In essence, we are now grappling with the repercussions of their poor eating habits. Astonishingly, studies have demonstrated that the disruptions caused by food chemicals can extend up to three generations—a genuinely eye-opening phenomenon!

What is the fuzz with pesticides and herbicides?

In today's world, agriculture plays an important role in sustaining human life. However, the use of pesticides and herbicides in farming practices has raised concerns and questions. The complexities and potentially harmful effects surrounding these chemicals shed light on their impact on our environment and health.

Pesticides are chemicals or substances that kill, repel, or control pests, including insects, weeds, fungi, rodents, and other organisms. They are crucial in modern agriculture and public health efforts to prevent disease vectors.

Benefits and Risks: Pesticides offer several benefits in agriculture, public health, and pest control. However, it's crucial to be aware of the potential risks associated with their use.

Pesticides Risks

Environmental Impact: Pesticides can have unintended effects on non-target organisms, including beneficial insects, birds, and aquatic life. They can disrupt ecosystems and contribute to biodiversity loss.

Residue Buildup: Pesticide residues can accumulate in the environment, potentially leading to long-term environmental contamination. They can persist in soil, water, and plants from a few months to 4 years or more.

Pesticide Resistance: Pests can develop resistance to pesticides over time, making them less effective. This can lead to the need for stronger or more frequent applications, which can exacerbate environmental risks.

Human Health Concerns

Pesticide exposure can pose risks to human health, particularly for those who handle or are exposed to high levels of these chemicals. This includes farmers, farmworkers, and individuals living near treated areas. Pesticides infiltrate the food chain through a multitude of avenues. The initial application of pesticides onto crops is a common entry point. These chemicals, intended to safeguard the plants from pests, may become integrated into the plant tissue. The integration of pesticides into plant tissue and subsequent consumption by livestock can lead to the accumulation of these chemicals in the animal's body. This, in turn, can result in pesticide residues in animal-derived products such as meat, milk, and eggs. Humans can potentially be exposed to these residues when they consume these products.

Furthermore, environmental factors come into play. Rainfall, for instance, carries remnants of pesticides from treated fields. This runoff can transport these chemicals into nearby streams and water bodies, initiating a chain reaction. Plankton (the microscopic organisms that form the basis of aquatic food chains) readily absorb these pesticide residues. As larger organisms feed on plankton, the pesticides ascend through the trophic levels. So, the process continues as small fish and invertebrates consume the contaminated plankton. As they, in turn, become prey for larger species, the pesticides ascend through the hierarchy of the aquatic ecosystem. Eventually, these chemicals reach fish of interest for human consumption, effectively entering the human food chain.

This process is a crucial consideration in the broader environmental and human health context. It underscores the need for meticulous management and vigilant strategies to mitigate the potential risks associated with pesticide use in agriculture. This comprehensive understanding of pesticide entry into the food chain is pivotal for establishing sustainable and responsible practices in modern agriculture and environmental conservation. This highlights the need for careful pesticide management and monitoring throughout the agricultural and food production process to ensure the safety of the food supply chain. The widespread presence of pesticides within various tiers of the food chain raises critical concerns about their potential impact on ecosystems and human health. Understanding these pathways is essential for developing strategies to mitigate the risks associated with pesticide use in agriculture and environmental management.

Yet, this glaring lapse in regulatory responsibility has left the public exposed to potential risks. Regrettably, the institutions charged with ensuring our safety have fallen short of their duty. It raises the pressing question of whose interests are indeed being prioritized. We must hold these authorities accountable and demand a thorough reevaluation of their practices. Our collective safety should never be compromised for any agenda other than the well-being of the public they serve. It's time for a systemic change that places public health and safety as their priorities.

The failure of the authorities entrusted with oversight is glaringly evident. Their duty to regulate these chemicals and ensure public safety has been neglected. It appears that these authorities' priorities are not concerned with public welfare. Instead, they seem swayed by alternative agendas, leaving the population vulnerable to the potential hazards posed by these harmful chemicals. This calls for a critical reevaluation of the regulatory framework and a demand for greater accountability in safeguarding the population's well-being.

Drift and Runoff: Pesticides can drift from their intended application site, potentially affecting neighboring areas or water bodies. Runoff can carry pesticides into waterways, posing risks to aquatic life.

Potential for Misuse: Pesticides can be ineffective or cause unintended harm if not used according to label instructions. This includes applying them at the wrong time, using incorrect doses, or ignoring safety precautions.

Groundwater Contamination: Some pesticides have the potential to leach through the soil and contaminate groundwater, posing risks to drinking water sources.

Regulatory Challenges: Proper pesticide use regulation and oversight can be challenging, especially in regions with limited resources or where enforcement is not enhanced.

Balancing the benefits and risks of pesticide use requires careful consideration of factors such as application methods, dosage, timing, and selecting less-toxic alternatives whenever possible. Integrated Pest Management (IPM) approaches aim to minimize the risks associated with pesticide use by incorporating a range of pest control strategies. This may include biological controls, cultural practices, and resistant crop varieties.

Insecticides are designed to kill or control insects. They can target specific types of insects or have a broader spectrum of activity.

Herbicides are designed to control or kill unwanted plants, commonly known as weeds. They can be non-selective (killing a wide range of plants) or selective (targeting specific types of plants, like broadleaf weeds or grasses).

Fungicides are used to control or prevent fungal diseases in crops, ornamental plants, and other agricultural settings. They work by inhibiting the growth and reproduction of fungi.

Rodenticides are used to control rodents such as mice, rats, and other small mammals. They can be lethal or act as growth regulators, affecting rodents' reproductive capabilities.

Bactericides control harmful bacteria in agricultural settings, particularly in the production of fruits, vegetables, and ornamental plants. They also help prevent bacterial diseases.

Nematicides are used to control nematodes, microscopic, worm-like organisms that can harm plants. They are commonly used in agriculture to protect crops.

Avicides are used to control birds, particularly in agricultural settings where they may threaten crops. They can be used to deter or reduce bird populations.

Molluscicides control mollusks, such as slugs and snails, that can damage crops and ornamental plants; they are often used in gardens and agricultural settings.

Piscicides are used to control fish populations, often in situations where certain fish species are considered invasive or harmful to native ecosystems.

Repellents are substances designed to deter pests without necessarily killing them. They are commonly used to keep insects, animals, and birds away from specific areas.

Attractants are substances used to lure pests into traps or bait stations, making it easier to control them without using more extensive pesticide applications.

Biopesticides are derived from natural materials, such as plants, bacteria, or fungi, and are considered environmentally friendly alternatives to synthetic chemical pesticides. They include substances like neem oil, insecticidal soaps, and beneficial insects.

Desiccants are substances that cause rapid drying of plants or pests, often used when fast desiccation is desirable.

Environmental Implications of Pesticides

The use of pesticides can have various environmental implications, both immediate and long-term. Here are some of the key environmental concerns associated with pesticide use:

Non-Target Species: Pesticides are designed to target specific pests, but they can also affect non-target species. Beneficial insects, such as bees and ladybugs, can be harmed by pesticide exposure. This disrupts natural predator-prey relationships and can lead to imbalances in ecosystems.

Biodiversity Loss: Pesticides can have widespread effects on biodiversity. They can harm non-target plants, insects, birds, and aquatic life. This can lead to declines in populations of various species, disrupt ecosystems, and potentially lead to long-term biodiversity loss.

Water Contamination: Pesticides can leach into groundwater or be carried by runoff into surface water bodies like rivers, lakes, and streams. This contamination poses risks to aquatic life and can affect water quality. Some pesticides can persist in water bodies for extended periods, leading to prolonged environmental impact. Contamination of groundwater by pesticides is a matter of national significance due to its role as a primary source of drinking water for roughly half of the nation's population. This is especially critical in agricultural regions, where pesticide usage is most prevalent, and approximately 95 percent of the inhabitants rely on groundwater for their drinking supply. Previously, it was believed that soil functioned as a barrier, preventing pesticides from infiltrating groundwater. However, research has dispelled this notion. Pesticides can now be traced to underground aquifers through various means, including field applications, tainted surface water, unintended spills, improper disposal, and even the injection of waste materials into wells.

Soil Degradation: Pesticides can alter soil health and composition. They may disrupt the balance of beneficial microorganisms in the soil, affecting nutrient cycling and potentially reducing soil fertility. Prolonged use of certain pesticides can contribute to soil degradation.

Residue Buildup: Pesticide residues can accumulate in the environment over time. These residues may persist in soil, water, and plants, potentially leading to long-term environmental contamination. This can pose risks to both terrestrial and aquatic ecosystems.

Pesticide Drift: During application, pesticides can drift away from the target area due to factors like wind. This can result in unintended exposure to non-target plants and animals. Pesticide drift can also lead to contamination of nearby crops, affecting both agricultural and natural ecosystems.

Wildlife Exposure: Wildlife that inhabits areas treated with pesticides can be directly exposed to these chemicals. This exposure can lead to acute toxicity or have sub-lethal effects, impacting behavior, reproduction, and overall health.

Development of Pesticide Resistance: Over time, pests can develop resistance to pesticides. This occurs when individuals with natural resistance traits survive pesticide exposure and pass on these traits to their offspring. This can render certain pesticides ineffective, leading to the need for stronger or more frequent applications.

Secondary Pest Outbreaks: Pesticides can disrupt natural predator-prey relationships, leading to outbreaks of secondary pests. When predators are reduced or eliminated, populations of other pests can increase, potentially leading to the need for additional pesticide applications.

Air Quality Impact

Pesticides applied as sprays or dusts can become airborne, potentially affecting air quality. This can affect human health, particularly for individuals near treated areas. When pesticides are applied in the form of sprays or dusts, they have the potential to become airborne, meaning that the pesticide particles can be carried by the wind and dispersed over a larger area beyond the intended target. This can lead to respiratory issues, especially for individuals with pre-existing conditions like asthma or chronic obstructive pulmonary disease (COPD). Even for those without existing respiratory conditions, exposure to airborne pesticides can irritate the nose, throat, and lungs.

Exposure to Harmful Chemicals: Pesticides often contain chemicals that, when inhaled, can harm human health. Long-term exposure to certain pesticides has been associated with a range of health issues, including neurological effects, reproductive problems, and an increased risk of certain cancers. Children, older adults, and individuals with compromised immune systems are particularly vulnerable to the health effects of airborne pesticides. Their bodies may have a more challenging time metabolizing and eliminating these chemicals. Due to the potential risks associated with airborne pesticides, regulatory agencies often establish guidelines and restrictions regarding pesticide application methods, including wind speed and weather conditions. These measures are designed to minimize the potential for airborne drift.

Pesticides Benefits

Increased Crop Yields: Pesticides protect crops from pests, diseases, and weeds, which can result in more efficient food production. This helps meet the demands of a growing global population.

Reduced Economic Losses: Pest control keeps many crops safe from pests and diseases. Pesticides help minimize these losses, ensuring economic stability for farmers.

Public Health Protection: Pesticides are crucial in controlling disease vectors like mosquitoes and ticks, helping prevent the spread of diseases like malaria, Zika virus, and Lyme disease.

Improved Livestock Health: Pesticides are used to control parasites and diseases that can affect livestock, leading to healthier animals and higher-quality animal products.

Enhanced Aesthetic Value: Pesticides are used in landscaping and ornamental horticulture (to maintain the appearance and health of lawns, gardens, and public spaces).

Food Safety: Pesticides help ensure that food products are safe for consumption by reducing the presence of harmful pathogens and contaminants.

Pesticides and herbicides are crucial tools in modern agriculture, but their use requires careful consideration of their benefits and risks. Striking a balance between meeting the demands of a growing population and ensuring environmental sustainability is vital for human health. By exploring alternative pest control methods and advocating for responsible practices, we can pave the way for a more sustainable agricultural future, leading to healthier humans that can prevent diseases linked with pesticide exposures.

It's important to note that while pesticides can be practical tools for pest control, they should be used with care and according to label instructions to minimize environmental impact and potential harm to non-target organisms.

The role of consumers in pesticide management and environmental protection is vital. As a consumer, you can educate yourself about the products you regularly purchase. This includes understanding where their food comes from, how it's grown, and whether pesticides are used. Opting for organic or sustainably produced goods can reduce the demand for conventionally grown products with higher pesticide residues.

Supporting Sustainable Practices: By choosing products from companies and farmers who prioritize sustainable and eco-friendly practices, consumers create a market demand for these alternatives. This encourages more producers to adopt environmentally responsible approaches.

Advocacy for Regulation: As a consumer, you can influence policies and regulations. You can engage with local and national authorities to advocate for stricter regulations on pesticide use, better enforcement, and more transparent labeling.

Promoting Integrated Pest Management (IPM): As a consumer, you can support agricultural practices that focus on IPM. This approach emphasizes natural pest control methods and minimal use of pesticides, ultimately reducing their environmental impact. This holistic approach to pest management focuses on the long-term prevention of pests through biological control, habitat manipulation, modification of cultural practices, and use of resistant varieties. It minimizes the use of pesticides.

Reducing Waste and Pollution: Proper disposal of household pesticides, such as insecticides and herbicides, is crucial. Consumers should follow recommended guidelines and utilize hazardous waste facilities to prevent these chemicals from entering the environment.

Raising Awareness: As a consumer, you play a crucial role in spreading awareness about the impacts of pesticides on the environment and human health. By sharing information and advocating for change, you can influence a broader audience to open their eyes and be aware of the dangers associated with these harmful pesticides.

Personal Health Choices: You can also minimize personal exposure to pesticides such as washing fruits and vegetables thoroughly, using natural pest control methods in your home and gardens, and avoiding direct contact with chemical pesticides.

Monitoring and Reporting: If you suspect improper pesticide use or contamination, you should report it to the relevant authorities. This helps in identifying and addressing issues promptly.

By actively participating in these ways, you can, as a consumer, contribute significantly to reducing the environmental impact of pesticides and promoting sustainable, eco-friendly practices in agriculture and pest management.

Understanding Labels: Reading and understanding pesticide labels is essential. Labels provide information on the correct application, dosage, and safety precautions. It also indicates potential hazards to humans, animals, and the environment.

Professional Help: For complex pest issues, consider consulting a pest management professional who is trained in integrated pest management strategies.

Supporting Sustainable Agriculture is a crucial step towards a more environmentally friendly and resilient food system. By being informed and adopting responsible pesticide use practices, individuals can contribute to a healthier, safer, and more sustainable environment for themselves and future generations.

Buy Organic: Whenever possible, choose organic produce and products. Organic farming practices prioritize soil health, biodiversity, and natural pest management techniques.

Support Local Farmers: Purchase from local farmers' markets or subscribe to Community Supported Agriculture (CSA) programs. This reduces the carbon footprint associated with long-distance food transportation.

Reduce Food Waste: Minimize food waste by planning meals, using leftovers creatively, and composting organic waste, reducing the demand for excessive agricultural production.

Choose Seasonal Foods: Choose seasonal fruits and vegetables to support more natural growing cycles and reduce the need for energy-intensive greenhouse production.

Advocate for Sustainable Policies: Support policies and initiatives promoting sustainable agriculture, such as funding organic farming research, conservation programs, and incentives for sustainable practices.

Learn About Food Labels: Understand food labels like "organic," "non-GMO," and certifications from organizations like Fair Trade. These labels indicate products that adhere to specific sustainable practices.

Practice Home Gardening: If possible, grow your fruits, vegetables, and herbs. Even a small garden can reduce the demand for industrially produced crops.

Reduce Meat Consumption: Consider reducing meat consumption or adopting an intermittent or permanent plant-based diet. Livestock agriculture has a significant environmental footprint, including land use, water consumption, and greenhouse gas emissions.

Educate Yourself and Others: Stay informed about sustainable agriculture practices and share this knowledge with your friends, family, and social media community. Education is a powerful tool for driving positive change.

Engage with Sustainable Brands: Support companies that prioritize sustainable sourcing and production practices. Look for certifications like Rainforest Alliance, Fair Trade, and USDA Organic.

Participate in Community Gardens: Community gardening projects can be a transformative and empowering experience for individuals and neighborhoods. These spaces contribute to local food production and create a sense of community, unity, and shared purpose. They serve as valuable educational platforms, offering insights into sustainable agriculture practices, from seed planting to harvest. If your community doesn't have a gardening project, don't hesitate to take the initiative, and start one. Begin by seeking the necessary permits and permissions from local authorities and ensuring compliance with regulations or guidelines, and this might involve conversations with municipal officials, zoning boards, or community organizations.

The journey of community gardening is not just about growing plants; it's about nurturing relationships, cultivating a sense of belonging, and creating the seeds of sustainable living. It's a collective effort that enriches the environment and strengthens your community. So, whether you're tending to a small plot or a thriving garden, every contribution counts towards a greener, more connected, and sustainable future. Advocacy and policy play crucial roles in promoting sustainable agriculture and shaping the future of our food systems.

Promoting Sustainable Farming Practices

Advocacy efforts can focus on encouraging and incentivizing farmers to adopt sustainable practices like crop rotation, agroforestry, and integrated pest management to improve soil health and biodiversity and reduce environmental impacts.

Research and Innovation Funding: Advocacy groups can advocate for increased government funding for research and innovation in sustainable agriculture, which could lead to the development of new technologies and practices that benefit farmers and the environment.

Supporting Local Food Systems: Policies can be enacted to support local food systems, such as providing grants or tax incentives for small-scale, sustainable farming operations to help reduce the reliance on large-scale, industrial agriculture.

Regulating Pesticide and Chemical Use: Advocacy efforts can push for stricter regulations on pesticides and harmful chemicals in agriculture to help protect the environment and human health.

Promoting Organic and Agroecological Farming: Advocacy groups can work to promote organic and agroecological farming methods through education, outreach, and policy initiatives for more sustainable and regenerative farming practices.

Addressing Food Security and Access: Advocacy can focus on policies that address food security issues, such as supporting initiatives that provide access to fresh, locally produced foods in underserved communities.

Climate Resilience and Adaptation: Advocacy efforts can push for policies that help farmers adapt to climate change, such as providing resources for climate-resilient farming practices and infrastructure.

Advocating for Fair Trade Practices: Supporting policies that promote fair trade practices can ensure that farmers receive reasonable prices for their products and are not exploited in the global market.

Education and Outreach Programs: Advocacy groups can work to implement educational programs that teach farmers about sustainable practices and provide them with the resources they need to transition to more sustainable farming methods.

Advocacy for Land Conservation and Restoration: Policies that protect and restore natural habitats and biodiversity can be advocated for, which are essential components of sustainable agricultural systems.

Collaboration and Networking: Advocacy efforts can involve partnerships between farmers, researchers, policymakers, and community organizations to create a collective approach to sustainable agriculture.

Monitoring and Accountability: Advocacy groups can advocate for transparent monitoring and reporting of agricultural practices and their environmental impacts, enabling better accountability.

Advocacy and policy initiatives are essential for driving positive change in the agricultural sector toward more sustainable and regenerative practices. We can work towards a more resilient and environmentally friendly food system by advocating for policies that prioritize sustainability.

FAQs about Pesticides and Herbicides

Are all pesticides harmful to humans?
While pesticides are designed to target specific pests, some can pose risks to humans.

What are some natural alternatives to herbicides?
Natural alternatives like mulching, hand weeding, and using beneficial insects can be effective in controlling weeds without the use of chemical herbicides.

How do herbicide-resistant crops affect farming practices?
Herbicide-resistant crops allow farmers to use specific herbicides to control weeds without harming the crop to more efficient and sustainable farming practices.

How can consumers reduce their exposure to pesticide residues?

Washing fruits and vegetables thoroughly, buying organic produce, and supporting integrated pest management practices can help reduce pesticide residues in food.

What role do genetically modified crops play in pesticide use?

Genetically modified crops, including those with built-in pest resistance, can help reduce the need for external pesticide applications. However, their long-term effects are still a subject of ongoing research and discussion.

Accessing information about products and their manufacturers has never been easier in today's interconnected world. Beyond just a phone number, many companies maintain comprehensive websites that serve as information hubs. These sites often feature detailed product descriptions, ingredient lists, usage instructions, and customer reviews. Moreover, socially responsible companies frequently go the extra mile, providing insights into their manufacturing processes, sourcing practices, and sustainability initiatives. This transparency demonstrates a commitment to quality and highlights a dedication to consumer trust and satisfaction. By taking advantage of these resources, consumers like you have the power to make informed choices that align with your values and preferences. This level of access empowers individuals to support businesses that prioritize ethics, quality, and transparency, ultimately promoting a marketplace where integrity and accountability thrive.

So, when you invest your hard-earned money in a product, you are not just making a purchase but endorsing a brand that values your trust and well-being. This symbiotic relationship between consumers and responsible companies forms the foundation of a healthy, sustainable marketplace.

Storytime: Nourishing the Temple-A Journey to Wholesome Living

In the bustling of modern life, amidst the whirlwind of responsibilities and commitments, there exists a quiet sanctuary – the Anatomical House, or AnaHo, as we fondly call it. It is within this intricate dwelling that the delicate dance of life unfolds. We provide our bodies with sustenance daily, shaping our vitality and well-being.

Within AnaHo, the symphony of nutrients plays an important role. Fresh fruits and vegetables, gleaming with vibrant colors, are our truest allies. They are not merely food but life's elixir, granting us with nature's purest gifts. Yet, the journey towards wholesome living can be complicated. In a world where convenience often trumps nutrition, it's easy to fall prey to quick fixes and processed fare.

In AnaHo's embrace, we learn that every healthy food bite is a message to our cells, a pledge to nurture the inner universe. This profound understanding transcends taste alone. We recognize that nourishing ourselves is an act of self-respect, a promise to honor the sanctity of our bodies.

Through seasons and times, AnaHo remains our companion. We grasp the significance of portion control and the art of mindful eating. We understand that it is not only what we eat but how and when we do so that shapes our journey. With each plate, we become architects of our well-being.

As we explore meal preparation, we discover the beauty of balance. We learn to freeze with care, preserving both flavor and nutrients. The frozen treasures await their turn, providing us with sustenance, delight, and wisdom of mindful meal planning.

In this sanctuary, we acknowledge the whispers of our bodies, learning to decipher their cravings to distinguish true hunger from mere appetite. We learn to cherish eating as a sacred ritual, a communion with ourselves and the nourishment provided by the Earth.

Through the seasons of our lives, we walk this path of wholesome living, understanding that our bodies are not mere machines but temples to be revered. Each day is an opportunity to honor the miracle of life, to nourish and cherish, and to forge a harmonious union with AnaHo, the sacred abode that sustains us all. The end!

Journaling Time

1. What health goals do you want to achieve, and why are they important to you?

_____

_____

_____

_____

2. How does your current lifestyle align with your optimal health and wellness vision?

_____

_____

_____

_____

3. What habits, whether positive or negative, have the most significant impact on your well-being?

_____

_____

_____

_____

4. What role does mental and emotional health play in your wellness?

_____

_____

5. Are there any recurring patterns or behaviors holding you back from better health?

_____
_____
_____

6. How does your environment, including your home, workplace, and community, support or hinder your wellness goals?

_____
_____
_____

7. What are your primary sources of motivation and inspiration for maintaining a healthy lifestyle?

_____
_____
_____

8. How do you approach challenges and setbacks in your journey toward better health?

_____
_____
_____

9. Are there specific changes you have considered improving your well-being but have yet to implement?

_____
_____
_____

10. What steps can you take today to prioritize your health and make positive changes?

You can achieve remarkable things. Believe in yourself! You can do it! Your health is the foundation upon which you can build a life of vibrancy, purpose, and fulfillment. Every small choice to support your well-being is a step towards a brighter future.

You hold the power to transform your life, to write a story of vitality, and to inspire those around you. Never underestimate the positive impact your journey can have on others. Keep moving forward, one step at a time. Celebrate your progress and be compassionate with yourself when faced with challenges. Know that every effort you invest in your health is a profound act of self-love.

You can nourish your body, mind, and soul with each sunrise. Cherish this gift, and let it fuel your pursuit of a life lived in fullness. Your healthy journey is not a destination; it's a lifelong adventure. Embrace it with open arms, and may it lead you to a future of boundless vitality and joy. Thank you for allowing me to be a part of your journey.

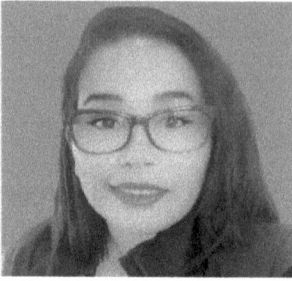

About the Author:

Meet Solanyi, an exceptional Nurse Consultant and Transformational Coach with a mission to empower individuals to lead healthier and happier lives, both physically and mentally. With over a decade of experience in the healthcare industry, Solanyi has witnessed firsthand the detrimental effects of unhealthy habits on the mind, body, and soul.

Driven by her passion for wellness, Solanyi created The Guided Route to Wellness, a robust platform that has positively impacted countless lives worldwide. Her extensive knowledge and expertise inspire individuals to take charge of their health, prevent diseases. Solanyi specializes in disease prevention and provides crucial tools and mindsets to avoid diseases. For those with chronic illnesses, she offers a framework for effective management and prevention of illness-related complications.

In a world where preventable diseases are rampant, Solanyi invites you to seize the opportunity to transform your life radically. Say goodbye to mediocrity and embrace a life of vibrant health, boundless energy, and unshakeable happiness. Solanyi is a fearless advocate for empowering individuals to lead positive, fulfilling, and joyful lives. Let her equip you with essential tools and a transformative mindset and revolutionize your life with exuberant health, boundless energy, and happiness.

For book references and additional resources, please visit:
http://grwcoaching.com

Once on the website, click the menu tab and select **HOD Nurturing the Universe Within.**

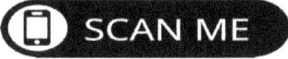

www.ingramcontent.com/pod-product-compliance
Lightning Source LLC
Chambersburg PA
CBHW062123020426
42335CB00013B/1070